Manual of Cooperative Group Treatment for Aphasia

Manual of Cooperative Group Treatment for Aphasia

Jan R. Avent, Ph.D.
Associate Professor of Communicative Sciences and Disorders, California State University, Hayward

Butterworth–Heinemann

Boston•Oxford•Johannesburg•Melbourne•New Delhi•Singapore

Recognizing the importance of preserving what has been written, Butterworth–Heinemann prints its books on acid-free paper whenever possible.

 Butterworth–Heinemann supports the efforts of American Forests and the Global ReLeaf program in its campaign for the betterment of trees, forests, and our environment.

Library of Congress Cataloging-in-Publication Data

Manual of cooperative group treatment for aphasia / [edited by] Jan R. Avent.
  p. cm.
  Includes bibliographical references and index.
  ISBN 0-7506-9921-3 (alk. paper)
  1. Aphasia--Treatment. 2. Group psychotherapy. 3. Group work in education. I. Avent, Jan R.
  [DNLM: 1. Aphasia--therapy. WL 340.5 M294 1997]
RC425.M27 1997
616.85'5206--dc21
DNLM/DLC
for Library of Congress   97-21508
                         CIP

British Library Cataloguing-in-Publication Data
A catalogue record for this book is available from the British Library.

The publisher offers discounts on bulk orders of this book.
For information, please contact:
Manager of Special Sales
Butterworth–Heinemann
313 Washington Street
Newton, MA 02158–1626
Tel: 617-928-2500
Fax: 617-928-2620

For information on all B–H publications available, contact our World Wide Web home page at http://www.bh.com

10 9 8 7 6 5 4 3 2 1

Printed in the United States of America

To our clients, who continue to teach us about aphasia and its treatment

Contents

Contributing Authors

Jan R. Avent, Ph.D.
Associate Professor of Communicative Sciences and Disorders, California State University, Hayward

Laura H. Fisher, M.S.
Speech-Language Pathologist, Communication Learning Network, Davis, California

Penny Hatch, M.S.
Speech-Language Pathologist, Alameda Unified School District, Alameda, California

Elizabeth L. Hoover, M.S.
Speech-Language Pathologist, Davies Medical Center, San Francisco

Susan Klingman, M.S.
Speech-Language Pathologist, Central California Rehabilitation Hospital, Modesto, California

Preface

In 1991, I attended the first of many workshops on cooperative learning in an attempt to improve my classroom teaching skills. It didn't take long for my "clinician's brain" to see the potential of cooperative learning as a treatment for aphasia. As I began implementing cooperative group treatment, my enthusiam for it grew. I tried various steps, materials, measures of treatment outcome, and numbers of participants. What worked remained and what didn't work was discarded or modified. Some of my groups were similar in language severity, while others were mixed. Some of the groups consisted of individuals with head injury and aphasia; other groups were entirely aphasic or head-injured. I have trained dozens of graduate students in implementing cooperative group treatment or one of its variations. This book is about what I have learned about group treatment for aphasia using cooperative learning methods.

I have had many years of experience conducting both individual and group treatments for aphasia. Yet none of my previous experiences prepared me for the dynamic nature of group treatment conducted from a cooperative learning standpoint. The essence of this treatment is that it relies on mutually benenficial interactions between two brain-injured individuals. The clinician structures the framework for these interactions and then gradually withdraws support as the clients take more responsibility for their own treatment.

As a clinician, I am often impressed with the spirit and courage of many individuals with aphasia. They somehow cope with their communication difficulties and strive to communicate better. When it would be easier to avoid communication, they seek to participate. It is this spirit to participate that makes cooperative group treatment come alive. No two therapy sessions are alike, and in many ways, the treatment becomes a journey of discovery. The clients learn about aphasia from each other and develop skills to help themselves, and the clinician learns to turn over "the reins of treatment" to the group.

This book is a compilation of five clinicians' understanding of cooperative learning as applied to group treatment. The goal of the book is to provide a rationale and framework for cooperative group treatment, practical illustrations of treatment, and suggestions for additional cooperative group activities.

J.R.A.

Acknowledgments

I am indebted to three people who have influenced me in my approach to group treatments for aphasia. The person to whom I am grateful above all is Delaina Walker-Batson, who has taught me the importance of treating aphasia at the impairment, disability, and handicap levels. I am also indebted to her colleagues at the Dallas Aphasia Center, Sandra Curtis and Jean Ford, for many conversations about group treatments.

Many people at my university removed obstacles and encouraged me during the conceptualization and completion of this book. I am particularly grateful to the clinic coordinators Barbara Rockman and Shelley Simrin. They supported my efforts to develop this treatment in our clinic.

Finally, I would like to extend a special thanks to Dave Rossetti for teaching me "to pick a pace I can do all day." This philosophy passes the "Sparky Test."

Manual of Cooperative Group Treatment for Aphasia

1

Introduction to Cooperative Group Treatment

Jan R. Avent

Group therapy for aphasia evolved out of a need to provide services for the large number of head-injured veterans returning from World War II.[1] It continues to be viewed by many clinicians as an adjunct to individual treatment, but the appeal of group treatment is growing due to a variety of factors. First, results of recent investigations indicate that socially oriented group therapy can be effective in improving aphasic individuals' communication skills.[2-4] Second, health care reform creates the need for more group therapy as a means of providing treatment for a large number of aphasic individuals who are ineligible for costly individual treatment. Third, the impact of aphasia extends beyond linguistic factors and includes psychosocial issues,[5] such as interpersonal interactions and intrapersonal perspectives.[6] These psychosocial problems include increased depression, social isolation, loss of work, reduced leisure activities, restricted social life, loss of confidence, and overall decreases in life satisfaction.[5, 7, 8] Due to the far-reaching effects of aphasia, group treatments are appealing, because language impairments can be treated in a social context in which intrapersonal and interpersonal factors can be used to improve feelings of competency, adequacy, and self-esteem.[5, 8-10]

Cooperative group treatment[11] was developed to address both the psychosocial and communicative impairments of aphasia. It is based on cooperative learning principles. *Cooperative learning* is the instructional use of small groups that allow individuals to work together to maximize their learning and each other's learning.[12] In group situations, learning occurs because group members share information, work cooperatively on tasks, and explore each others' attitudes, opinions, and beliefs through group processes.[13] Group interactions that occur during cooperative learning include interactions among cognitive, affective, metacognitive, and social activities of the learners involved.[14] Therefore, the benefits of cooperative learning include shared goals and purposes, mutual interest among group members, better quality of work, better generalization of learning, improved feelings of self-esteem, and a greater ability to understand the perspective of other individuals.[15, 16] Cooperative learning, a well-known group approach used in academic settings from kindergarten through college levels, has not been widely used in aphasia group treatment.

The purpose of this book is to describe this approach to group treatment for aphasia. This chapter describes the rationales and development of cooperative group treatment. Chapters 2 and 3 describe the application of cooperative group treatment to individuals with aphasia (Chapter 2) and head injury (Chapter 3). Chapter 4 describes an advanced form of cooperative group treatment that incorporates story-grammar elements. Chapter 5 describes a variation of cooperative group treatment developed for individuals with moderate aphasia. Chapter 6 provides examples of cooperative learning tasks that could be adapted to aphasia group treatment.

Rationales of Cooperative Group Treatment

Group Size

Cooperative group treatment is conducted in groups of two aphasic individuals and a speech-language pathologist. A two-person group is chosen, because the dyad is the basic relationship of human communication.[17, 18] Two-person groups increase the amount of commitment to the group, eliminate or minimize possible coalition relationships, provide a greater sense of camaraderie and belonging, and provide greater practice time in treatment. In a two-person group there is greater coordination among members, a greater division of tasks and specialization of functions, greater concern with and attentiveness to other group members, better quality of work, better understanding of communication among group members, greater friendliness and feelings of self-esteem and esteem for the work of the group, and a greater ability to understand someone else's perspective.

Treatment Goal

The purpose of treatment is to improve procedural and narrative discourse abilities in mildly impaired aphasic clients. These two tasks are chosen, because they provide sufficient information for discussion and represent information that could be used conversationally outside of treatment.

Partner Roles

In cooperative group treatment, the clients are assigned the roles of recaller and facilitator.[19] The recaller summarizes the target story. The facilitator cues, corrects, and adds deleted information during the recaller's retelling of the target story. These roles are alternated for each target story.

Clinician Roles

The clinician has three major roles during cooperative group treatment: organizing the session, enhancing group processing skills, and teaching cueing strategies. Organizing the session includes selecting appropriate stories for use in treatment, data collection of treatment outcome, and providing homework assignments. Another role is to provide a therapeutic climate for cooperative learning. Throughout cooperative group treatment, the clinician enhances group processing skills by teaching the clients how to become more autonomous by helping one another (Table 1-1). The goal of increased autonomy is accomplished by the clinician providing support for cooperative learning, giving advice and suggestions, summarizing, clarifying, probing and questioning, repeating and paraphrasing, interpreting and analyzing, and listening. During this treatment, the clinician facilitates cooperation by gradually becoming less directly involved in the interactions between the clients. The final role of the clinician is to teach the clients about cueing. During the first few sessions, the clinician actively teaches the group members about

Table 1-1. Cooperative Learning Skills Used in Cooperative Group Treatment

---

Positive interdependence

The clients work together to complete tasks during treatment.

Face-to-face promotive interaction

Each client assists, supports, and encourages the learning of the other client.

Individual accountability and personal responsibility

Each client receives feedback about his or her performance, and discusses how to assist improvement of each other

Collaborative skills

The clients develop skills to improve decision making, trust building, communication, and conflict management.

Group processing

The clients discuss how they are achieving their goals and maintaining effective working relationships.

---

cues—types of cues (i.e., verbal cues, visual cues, gestures, drawing, and writing), examples of cues (e.g., saying the initial sound, pointing to a word in the key word list, pantomiming a word, writing a word), how to cue, and when to cue. Over time, as the members become proficient in cueing, the clinician prompts the facilitator as necessary.

Explanation of Treatment

For group treatment to be cooperative, the following characteristics should be present: positive interdependence, face-to-face promotive interaction, individual accountability and personal responsibility, collaborative skills, and group processing.[16] These skills are described to the clients during the first session together and are outlined in Table 1-1.

Positive Interdependence

Positive interdependence occurs when clients believe that they are linked with others such that their success depends on the success of others in the group.[12] Cooperative group treatment improves narrative and procedural story telling. In this treatment, the clinician assigns a particular story, narrative or procedural, and requires the group members to agree on the key elements of the story. The number of key words and phrases selected per story, which is usually between eight and ten, and the amount of time used to complete the assignment is limited; therefore, groups must learn to select the best key elements, negotiate disagreements over key-word selection, and use time effectively.[11] Over time, groups learn strategies to improve key-word selection. For example, one strategy they generally develop is taking turns selecting key words.

Face-to-Face Promotive Interaction

Face-to-face promotive interaction occurs when the clients help, assist, encourage, and support each other's efforts to learn. Each client promotes his or her partner's learning by explaining rationales for problem solving, discussing the concepts to be remembered and learned, teaching his or her knowledge to the other, and explaining the connections between present and past learning.[11] For example, a target narrative story dealt with the sinking of the *Titanic*. One aphasic person consistently forgot the date of this disaster. Her partner taught her a strategy for remembering the date—that is, to associate the date with another important date. The aphasic individual associated 1912 with the year her mother was born. She never forgot the date after learning this strategy from her aphasic partner.

Individual Accountability

Individual accountability exists when each client's performance is assessed and the results are provided as feedback. With this type of feedback, the members learn to cue better, to ask for assistance when needed, and to develop strategies to improve performance.[11] The clinician provides three types of feedback during the session: number of key elements recalled in a 1-minute story retelling task performed with no facilitator help, number and type of facilitator-initiated cues during the practice portion of story retelling, and the number of recaller-initiated requests for assistance during story-recall practice. Following the feedback for each story, the aphasic partners and clinician discuss ways to improve performance (e.g., initial-sound cueing is better than spelling for some persons) and provide encouragement and reinforcement for effort and performance.

In addition to the within-treatment feedback, generalization data are collected on untreated stories. These probes are taken every fourth session and are used to monitor progress over time.

Group Processing

Group processing refers to the group members' ongoing discussions of the benefit of treatment, how the members can better work together, and how the group members can improve their effectiveness during cueing and key-word selection. For example, the clinician often asks the clients at the end of the session to discuss the cues that were helpful and those that were not helpful, to evaluate the story retelling task, and to suggest ways to make the treatment more beneficial.

Treatment Sequence

For each new story introduced in treatment, the following sequence occurs:

1. The clinician reads the story as the clients follow along with their copy of the story.

2. The clinician and clients review the story. The clients compile a list of eight to ten key words or short phrases about the story.

3. The recaller practices telling the story without the benefit of the story or key-word list. When cueing is needed, the facilitator provides specific cues. The clinician prompts the facilitator as necessary.

4. The recaller practices telling the story in about 1 minute. No cueing is provided.

5. The facilitator and clinician provide feedback to the recaller to improve performance. The recaller provides feedback to the facilitator about the appropriateness of the cues during cued recall.

6. At the end of the session, the clients and clinician discuss the session (debrief). They evaluate the stimulus stories, cueing, and performances of the recaller and facilitator, and discuss ways of making the treatment better.

Length of Treatment

Cooperative group treatment can be conducted in sessions that last from about 45 minutes (with one story per session) to 90 minutes (with two or three stories per session).

Treatment Outcome Measures

Various measures are sensitive to improvements that occur during cooperative group treatment. Improvements in the amount of information provided during story retelling is documented with the correct information unit analysis described by Nicholas and Brookshire.[20] Generalization is measured via the correct information units used in three stories, which are similar to those used in treatment or the pictures described in Nicholas and Brookshire. These generalization probes are administered to the clients individually every fourth session. During treatment, two simple scoring methods are used to provide clients with immediate feedback about their performance. First, a tally of the number of key words used by the recaller during a 1-minute story retelling is used to document improved relevant content of the treatment stories. Second, number and types of appropriate cues provided by the facilitator are tallied during the practice recall. Both of these measures—key words used during retelling and facilitator cues—can be discussed by the group when evaluating daily progress and reported in daily notes. At the end of treatment, a social validation questionnaire is used to evaluate treatment. Examples of social validation questionnaires are in Chapters 2, 4, and 5.

Essence of Cooperative Learning Groups

Group Cohesiveness Develops Over Time

All groups undergo a process of development, which includes relationship formation, stabilization, decision making, and evolving patterns of behavior.[13] Tuckman's model of the stages of development in a group is used to describe cooperative group treatment. His categories of forming, storming, norming, and performing[21] are used as a guide for documenting changes in the formation of each group over time and to assist the clinician in learning to implement this treatment.

In cooperative group treatment, the forming stage lasts from one to three sessions. Examples of this stage occur when members "size each other up," evaluate their resources and talents, learn task expectations, and determine how they will work together on their goals.[11] In this early stage, the group members generally seek the clinician's approval of key-word and phrase selection. The storming stage occurs during the third to fifth sessions. During this stage, members begin to have disagreements over key-word and phrase selection. When these conflicts occur, the group must learn how to deal with different opinions.[11] A common strategy to reduce conflicts during this stage is for members to agree to all key words that are selected. The norming stage occurs during the sixth to eighth sessions, with the members developing rules to govern their activities. During this stage, the group members learn to negotiate and discuss their choices before reaching a decision. The importance of this stage is that it is the beginning of cohesiveness.[11] Group members often disagree about key-word selection and must develop skills to negotiate joint decisions. The last stage, the performing stage, begins around the eighth or ninth session and characterizes the remainder of treatment.[11] During this stage, the members have developed strategies to resolve conflicts over key-word selection and are somewhat independent of the clinician. A list of behaviors observed during these stages is in Figure 1-1.

Key-Word Selection

A vital portion of cooperative group treatment is the selection of key words from each story. This activity requires cooperation between the group members, because both members benefit from the key words. That is, the recaller attempts to use all of the key words during story retelling and the facilitator uses the key words to cue the recaller.

There are no right answers when choosing key words, although some words are better than others. The ambiguity in key-word selection leads to improved decision-making skills, because the clients must discuss their word choices.[22] These discussions lead to improved oral summarizing, explaining, and elaboration of knowledge and opinions.[23] In other words, key-word selection is not a contrived task, but one that creates real dialogue for the authentic exchange of information.

Treatment Candidates

Language Impairment

Cooperative group treatment is designed for mildly impaired individuals with aphasia. It has been modified and applied to moderately impaired individuals (see Chapter 5) and used with high-level head-injured individuals (see Chapter 3). Cooperative group treatment is not recommended for severely impaired individuals with aphasia. Use of other cooperative learning procedures in the treatment of severe aphasia is possible, and many of the tasks described in Chapter 6 could be appropriately modified for group treatment of severe aphasia.

Group Formation Process: Observation Guide

Check specific behavior in the space provided. Document both positive and negative behaviors.

Clients' name: _____

Clinician's name: _____

Date: _____

Sessions	√	Skills	Comments
1 and 2	__	Clinician instructs and models all aspects of treatment	
	__	Clinician models most of cues	
	__	Eye contact mainly between client and clinician	
	__	Poor eye contact between partners	
	__	Little or no cooperation between partners	
	__	Talking between partners infrequent	
	__	No negotiation on key words, all suggestions accepted	
	__	Partners seek clinician input regarding key-word selection	
3 and 4	__	Negotiation beginning between partners	
	__	Increased concentration on tasks	
	__	Increased competence in key word compilation	
	__	Decreased reliance on clinician for key-word selection	
	__	Clinician continues to prompt facilitator cueing	
	__	Clinician continues to direct debriefing	

Figure 1-1. Observation guide of group formation behaviors during cooperative group treatment. (From JR Avent. Group treatment in aphasia using cooperative learning method. J Med Speech-Lang Pathol 1997;5:9.)

Sessions	√	Skills	Comments
4 and 5	__	Partners share personal information (e.g., the effects of aphasia)	
	__	Increased eye contact between partners	
	__	Increased reliance on partner, less reliance on clinician	
	__	Increased independence of facilitator to cue partner	
	__	Increased collaboration on key-word list	
	__	More opinions stated by partners to negotiate key words	
	__	Increased ease of interactions (e.g., more laughter, sharing)	
	__	Increased cooperation on tasks	
	__	Decreased clinician direction and control	
	__	Clinician continues to direct debriefing	
7 and above	__	Decreased clinician direction of debriefing	
	__	Increased partner participation (e.g., talking)	
	__	Increased use of questions between partners	
	__	Increased comments from partners about content of treatment	
	__	Increased amount of information shared between partners	
	__	Increased independence of partners during treatment	
	__	Clinician provides general directions as necessary	

Figure 1-1 (*continued*)

Reading Ability

Sentence-level and paragraph-level reading ability is ideal for cooperative group treatment but is not required. For clients who are moderately to mildly impaired and have limited reading ability, story pictures, such as sequential pictures or Norman Rockwell prints, can be used instead of written material.

Apraxia of Speech

Apraxia of speech can prevent some clients from fully participating in oral story retelling. For these individuals, communication notebooks are provided to improve communication skills. Story content and items for the communication notebook are selected based on client interest in various topics. Chapter 5 provides examples of the communication notebook approach.

Arrangement of Groups

Clients can be grouped randomly, based on similar language impairments, or by the interests of the members.[24] Cooperative group treatment has been implemented in groups in which clients have similar impairment levels and groups with different impairment levels.[11] Client improvements are possible in both types of groups. However, results of social validation questionnaires indicate that clients prefer a partner with similar language impairment. Gender and age differences do not appear to influence outcomes.

An additional consideration when grouping clients is the appropriate difficulty level of stimulus materials. In mixed language impairment groups, it is difficult, if not impossible, to select materials that are appropriate for both clients. Generally, materials appropriate for one client are either too easy or too difficult for the partner. Therefore, it is recommended that partners with similar language impairments be grouped (see the section on Different Language Severity Levels below).

Components of Group Treatment

According to Sampson and Marthas,[17] the two primary components of group treatment are the task and the process. The task is the outcome or productivity of the group, and the process refers to the cohesiveness of the group. One factor stands out in group treatment: The interactional portion becomes the primary function of the group and relates to the members' loyalty, pride, and commitment to the group. Throughout cooperative group treatment, the aphasic partners develop a special camaraderie. They discuss the impact of aphasia on their lives, describe an improved self-esteem that comes from helping someone else, and share a new-found willingness to socialize more in their daily lives. In many ways, the task, or the transactional portion of treatment, becomes a tool or a framework for these beneficial interactions.[11]

Research Results Using Cooperative Group Treatment

In 1997, I reported the results of a study using cooperative learning methods.[11] Eight aphasic subjects, mildly to moderately impaired, received cooperative group treatment. Two subjects were assigned to a treatment group following baseline measures for a total of four treatment groups.

A multiple baseline across behaviors within subject design was used to assess treatment and generalization effects.[25] The design involved two phases: baseline (i.e., the measure of performance before treatment) and treatment. Treatment was presented in sequence across time for two types of discourse: procedural and narrative. Treatment was conducted for about 18 sessions.

The results indicated that cooperative group treatment was effective in improving the content of narrative and procedural discourse in the mildly impaired aphasic subjects. In terms of language severity, all subjects who received pretreatment baseline performance scores of 20% or higher correct information units (CIU) per minute[20] and Western Aphasia Battery (WAB) Aphasia Quotient (AQ) scores above 75 improved with treatment and showed generalization effects. The remaining moderately impaired subjects with baseline performance scores below 20% correct information unit per minute and WAB AQ scores between 45 and 65 showed no treatment or generalization effects.

Problem Solving: What if Cooperative Learning Groups Are Not Working?

Team Building

Groups do not automatically work together efficiently. In the first session or two, it is helpful to establish a cohesive framework based on group processes. The most important group process characteristic at this stage of group work is group membership. Group membership is enhanced by learning the names of the team members, learning about the team members, and completing a cooperative activity together. To learn about team members, it is often helpful to provide name tags with a twist. On the name tag, include a piece of trivial information such as the person's town of residence, favorite food, number of children, or favorite movie star. To demonstrate the cooperative framework of the group, it is helpful to complete an activity that is difficult for an individual to complete alone (e.g., matching state capitals with states).

Potential Problems Within Groups

Failure to Get Along

Failure to get along often improves with time and after the group has some experience working cooperatively. In these situations, it is important for the clinician to be firm about the goal of treatment and to set guidelines for interactions. The clinician can also use social validation questionnaires at the end of treatment each day or weekly phone calls to clients, their "significant others," or both, to pinpoint problem areas, as well as solutions. In one instance, a client did not give her partner enough time to respond before cueing him. The clinician found out about the problem during a social validation questionnaire and helped the partner cue more appropriately. If groups are not working well after five or six sessions, it is best to switch partners.

Inappropriate Behavior

In some groups, clients become impatient with their partners, feel that their partner is talking too much, or wish to see their partner socially outside of treatment. With all of these scenarios, the clinician's duty is to refocus the session on the goals. Often, the clinician discusses specific inappropriate or distracting behaviors with the individual client in a private session and suggests possible solutions.

Absences

Absenteeism creates two problems: (1) The partner in treatment has no one to work with, and (2) the absent partner is missing important treatment time. For occasional absences, the clinician becomes the missing partner for that session and uses the time to practice cueing strategies through modeling and prompting. For the absent partner, homework activities are prepared for the material covered in the missed session and sent home for review. Chronic absenteeism is rare due to the cohesive nature of the groups. However, when it occurs, the chronic absentee is withdrawn from the cooperative treatment and a new partner is provided for the current client.

Ineffective Use of Team Practice Time

There is one primary problem that can result in ineffective use of team practice time. This problem is the clinician who dominates the practice time with suggestions, cues too much, provides feedback without client input, and so on. During cooperative group treatment, the clinician should monitor the session for signs of client passivity and should encourage the clients to help each other. If cueing or feedback is necessary, it should be provided indirectly by giving it to the facilitator partner and having that client help the recaller partner. The clinician should avoid giving feedback and cueing before prompting the clients to help each other.

Individual Practice

Some clients try to complete activities independently and appear to avoid helping or collaborating with their partner. There are a variety of solutions to try, which depend on the clients and the situation. One solution is to provide only one worksheet and one pencil. Another solution is to reinstruct on the process of cooperation. Scripting the interaction can be helpful. For example, insist that the clients take turns in completing the task; adding structure is often helpful.

Different Language Severity Levels

Given my experience with a variety of cooperative groups, I recommend avoiding groups with mixed severity levels. In mixed-severity groups, the team no longer works as peers but develops a mentor-student relationship that is not comfortable for either client. The more severely impaired client may feel that he or she is holding the partner back, and the less severely impaired person may feel that he or she is not getting quality practice time.

Different Treatment Goals

The group goal (e.g., improved content during story retelling) may be the same for each client, but specific goals may differ. Generally, the specific goals for each client are written down and reviewed at the beginning of the week or session. By stating the goals, each client can assist in helping his or her partner achieve these goals.

Number of Key Words

One of the essential elements in cooperative group treatment is the key-word selection process. To maximize discussions about key-word selections, it is important to limit the number of words that can be selected. If group members try to select more than ten words, the story may be too difficult, or the members may avoid negotiating over word choices. Either problem diminishes the rich interactions that can occur during key-word selection.

Poor Key-Word Selection

In some groups, particularly during the first few cooperative group treatment sessions, clients consistently choose key words that are not primary content words. There are several ways to improve key-word selection. One approach is to ask the clients to select one to two important words from each sentence. After the words are selected from each sentence, the clients review the list and select the ten most important words. Another approach is for the clinician to develop a key-word list independently of the clients. After the clients have selected their words, the two lists are compared and discussed. Following the discussion, the clients decide which key words to use. Another successful approach is to discuss the key words used during the 1-minute story retelling task and compare these words with the original list. This comparison often teaches the group members that some words are difficult to recall or are not important to the story. In this example, the group is encouraged to revise their list of key words and to try the story again.

Poor Cueing Skills

Learning how to cue a partner provides a framework for clients to learn self-cueing strategies. During treatment, the clinician teaches the group about cueing; however, some clients have difficulty learning to cue their partner. One suggestion is for the clinician to model an appropriate cue and ask the facilitator to provide that cue for their partner. While the modeling is redundant for the recaller, it often provides the necessary practice for the facilitator to learn cueing skills. Another suggestion is to collect a number of key words from different stories and ask the clients to practice cueing. One activity is to have a stack of cards with different cues (e.g., initial sound cue, rhyme, gesture, pantomime, draw, spell) and have one client draw a cue and provide an example of it with one of the key words.

Summary

Based on the results of research[11] and of other subsequent groups that have been treated, I continue to gain expertise in the implementation of cooperative learning groups. The remainder of this book is meant to be a guide. Each author presents her use of cooperative group treatment in the treatment of specific clients. The final chapter describes a variety of cooperative therapy approaches from the educational literature, with suggestions about how to adapt each approach to the treatment of aphasia.

References

1. Kearns KP. Group Therapy for Aphasia: Theoretical and Practical Considerations. In R Chapey (ed), Language Intervention Strategies in Adult Aphasia (3rd ed). Baltimore: Williams & Wilkins, 1994;304.
2. Wertz RT, Collins MJ, Weiss D, et al. Veterans Administration cooperative study on aphasia: A comparison of individual and group treatment. J Speech Hear Res 1981;24:580.
3. Aten JL, Caligiuri MP, Holland AL. The efficacy of functional communication therapy for chronic aphasic patients. J Speech Hear Disord 1982;47:93.
4. Elman R, Bernstein-Ellis E. Effectiveness of Group Communication for Individuals with Chronic Aphasia. Presented at the Seventh International Aphasia Rehabilitation Conference, Boston, August 1996.
5. Sarno MT. Aphasia rehabilitation: Psychosocial and ethical considerations. Aphasiology 1993;7:321.
6. Holland AL, Beeson PM. Finding a new sense of self: What the clinician can do to help. Aphasiology 1993;7:581.
7. Parr S. Coping with aphasia: Conversations with 20 aphasic people. Aphasiology 1994;8:457.
8. Le Dorze G, Brassard C. A description of the consequences of aphasia on aphasic persons and their relatives and friends based on the WHO model of chronic diseases. Aphasiology 1995;9:239.

9. Brumfitt S. Losing your sense of self: What aphasia can do. Aphasiology 1993;7:569.
10. Lyon J. Optimizing Communication and Participation in Life for Aphasic Adults and Their Prime Caregivers in Natural Settings: A Use Model for Treatment. In GL Wallace (ed), Adult Aphasia Rehabilitation. Boston: Butterworth–Heinemann, 1996;137.
11. Avent JR. Group treatment in aphasia using cooperative learning method. J Med Speech-Lang Pathol 1997;5:9.
12. Johnson DW, Johnson RT, Smith KA. Cooperative Learning: Increasing College Faculty Instructional Productivity. Washington, DC: George Washington University, School of Education and Human Development, 1991;1.
13. Davis JR. Better Teaching, More Learning: Strategies for Success in Postsecondary Settings. Phoenix: Oryx Press, 1993;242.
14. O'Donnell AM, Dansereau DF. Scripted Cooperation in Student Dyads: A Method for Analyzing and Enhancing Academic Learning and Performance. In R Hertz-Lazarowitz, N Miller (eds), Interaction in Cooperative Groups: The Theoretical Anatomy of Group Learning. New York: Cambridge University Press, 1992;120.
15. Deutsch M. A theory of cooperation and competition. Hum Rel 1949;2:129.
16. Slavin RE. Cooperative Learning: Theory, Research, and Practice. Boston: Allyn & Bacon 1995;1.
17. Sampson EE, Marthas MS. Group Process for the Health Professions. New York: Wiley, 1977;112.
18. Riccardi VM, Kurtz SM. Communication and Counseling in Health Care. Springfield, IL: Charles C. Thomas, 1983;211.
19. Larson CO, Dansereau DF. Cooperative learning in dyads. J Reading 1986;29:516.
20. Nicholas L, Brookshire RH. Quantifying connected speech of adults with aphasia. J Speech Hear Res 1993;36:338.
21. Tuckman BW. Developmental sequence in small groups. Psychol Bull 1965;63:384.
22. Samples R. Cooperation: Worldview as Methodology. In N Davidson, T Worsham (eds), Enhancing Thinking Through Cooperative Learning. New York: Teachers College Press, 1992;29.
23. Johnson DW, Johnson RT. Encouraging Thinking Through Constructive Controversy. In N Davidson, T Worsham (eds), Enhancing Think-

ing Through Cooperative Learning. New York: Teachers College Press, 1992;120.

24. Kagan S, Kagan M. The Structural Approach: Six Keys to Cooperative Learning. In S Sharan (ed), Handbook of Cooperative Learning Methods. Westport, CT: Greenwood, 1994;115.

25. McReynolds LV, Kearns KP. Single-Subject Experimental Designs in Communicative Disorders. Baltimore: University Park Press, 1983;51.

2

Cooperative Group Treatment for Individuals with Mild Aphasia

Susan Klingman

This chapter explores the use of cooperative group treatment to improve the verbal expression skills of individuals with mild aphasia. It describes the way the treatment approach was applied to two clients to increase the amount of information each client conveyed verbally during story recall tasks. Although these clients participated in a 2-month biweekly treatment program (for a total of eighteen 1-hour sessions), the approach could easily be adapted to accommodate other treatment schedules.

Determining Which Clients to Group

Several criteria were used to choose appropriate clients for the treatment dyad. The clients were matched according to

- *Classification of mild aphasia.* The classification of mild aphasia was determined from a current diagnosis of anomic aphasia for both clients using the Western Aphasia Battery (WAB).[1]

- *Specific language skills.* The verbal expression of both clients was marked by anomia in connected speech. Mild deficits in auditory comprehension were noted only for complex stimuli, such as multistep sequential commands. Both clients presented with reading and writing skills at the paragraph level.

• *Motivation.* Each client expressed interest in working with another individual in a group dyad setting. Both had worked diligently in earlier individual therapy to improve verbal expression skills and appeared motivated to continue improving verbal skills using this treatment approach.

• *Common interests.* The clients shared interests in professional football and travel. They were also approximately the same age and shared interests relating to their age cohort. These shared interests facilitated bonding during the initial stages of treatment.

Criteria that were not used in client selection included gender and etiology. The clients who were selected included a man, JG, who had a left-hemisphere cerebrovascular accident and a woman, LF, who had a left posterior cerebral artery aneurysm and subarachnoid hemorrhage followed by a left frontal craniotomy.

Baseline Assessment and Treatment Outcome Evaluation

Initial diagnostic testing was first performed, using the WAB,[1] to confirm the severity and type of aphasia. (The administration time was 60 minutes.) Baseline testing was then conducted to provide a measure of treatment outcome and to develop a plan for evaluating subsequent treatment sessions.

Assessment

All testing, including the initial diagnostic testing, was conducted for each client individually and was completed in two sessions per client (for a total of four of the 18 program sessions). To document overall treatment effects for improved naming, functional language, and story recall skills, the following tests and probes were helpful:

• Boston Naming Test[2] (administration time was 15–20 minutes).

• American Speech-Language Hearing Association Functional Assessment of Communication Skills for Adults[3] (no in-session administration time was required).

• Generalization probes (administration time was 10 minutes per testing session). To determine improvement in recall skills of similar stories used during the course of therapy, generalization probes of story recall tasks were used. Baseline performance levels were established by having the clients verbally recall two procedural and one narrative stories, similar to those planned for use during treatment. After listening to a story consisting of approximately 200 words, each client was asked to retell the story as completely as possible in 1 minute. The responses for each story were transcribed and analyzed for the percentage of correct information units (CIUs) per minute, using the method of Nicholas and Brookshire.[4] Three recall trials per client were conducted for each story to ensure consistency. Performance scores for each trial of the three stories were averaged to provide three baseline data points. The stories used were *Making Mashed Potatoes*, *Going Fishing*, and *Nile Crocodile* (see Appendix 2A).

Treatment Outcome Evaluation

Three methods were selected to measure improvement during the course of therapy: data collection during treatment sessions, administration of generalization probes, and collection of social validation data.

Daily Treatment Data Collection

Data were collected during each treatment session using score sheets (Figure 2-1). After reading a story, the clients agreed on ten key elements they thought were essential to the story. For scoring purposes, these were recorded by the clinician on the score sheet in the "Key Elements" column. The designated recaller then practiced retelling the story, while the facilitator provided cues. Data for this task were recorded in the two "Cued Recall" columns. Finally, the recaller attempted to retell the story without any cues from the partner, while the clinician scored correct responses in the "Recall Probe" column. All treatment steps mentioned—selecting key elements, cued recall, and the recall probe—are described in greater detail in following sections. Finally, on the bottom portion of the score sheet, the clinician transcribed, at a later time, all clinician, recaller, and facilitator cues and requests for assistance to track trends in cueing by using audio- or videotape recordings.

Score Sheet

Story: _____

Key Elements	Cued Recall Recaller: client 1 (√ = Without cue) (+ = With facilitator cue)	Cued Recall Facilitator: client 2 Cues provided:	Recall Probe Recaller: client 1 1-minute recall No cues provided (√ = Recall of key element)	Clinician Cues	Recaller Requests for Cues or Assistance	Facilitator Cues
1.						
2.						
3.						
4.						
5.						
6.						
7.						
8.						
9.						
10.						

◄ **Figure 2-1.** Score sheet used to record data for each story presented during treatment sessions. The top portion of the score sheet allows the clinician to record the ten key elements selected for the story (first column). The clinician records (1) whether the recaller recalls these key elements independently (√) or with cues from the facilitator (+) during cued recall (second column), (2) the cues the facilitator uses to help the recaller (third column), and (3) the key elements the recaller recalls (later converted to a percentage) during the 1-minute recall probe (fourth column). The bottom portion of the score sheet allows the clinician to transcribe from an audio- or videotape recording a complete record of cues used by the clinician and facilitator, along with all of the recaller's requests for cues. In this way the clinician can track trends in the clients' dependence on each other and decreases in dependence on the clinician for cues.

Bimonthly Generalization Probes

Bimonthly generalization probes consisted of the same three stories used to assess story recall skills during assessment. The two procedural stories, *Making Mashed Potatoes* and *Going Fishing*, were presented first and second, respectively, followed by the narrative story, *Nile Crocodile* (see Appendix 2A). Generalization probes were administered independently to each client once every other week until the completion of the treatment program. Each story was first presented verbally by the clinician, then recalled by the client. A picture of a crocodile was provided during each of the clinician's verbal presentations of *Nile Crocodile*. The entire three-story probe required approximately 10 minutes for administration. Each story was later transcribed from audiotape recordings and scored for CIUs. Another possible scoring technique is to select the most essential content and score the percentage of essential content recalled. No feedback about performance was provided during these probes.

Social Validation Data

Social validation data were gathered during each session and at the end of the program from responses recorded in the clients' journals, from discussions with the clients and their spouses, and from the clients' feedback on an end-of-treatment questionnaire. Questions posed to the clients and their spouses before and after treatment sessions yielded reports on improvements in communication skills outside of the clinical setting. These questions also involved spouses in the assessment of benefits of this treatment approach. A list of some questions that were helpful in soliciting social validation data from JG, LF, and their

Table 2-1. Sample of Questions Used to Elicit
Social Validation Data During Treatment

Did you do anything new or fun since we last met?

Have you faced any recent challenges in your life?

Have there been any changes in your activities?

How is this therapy helping you away from the clinic?

Have you felt different about your communication skills in any speaking
situation lately?

spouses is included in Table 2-1. An end-of-treatment questionnaire is
included as Figure 2-2.

Clinician's Task: Selecting Goals or Objectives for the Group

Quantifiable Goals

The following quantifiable goals were set for JG and LF:

1.   The primary goal for both members of the dyad was to improve
the content of their narrative and procedural discourse. This was measured by the number of key elements produced during recall probes,
recorded as a percentage, and by CIU scores on generalization probes.

2.   Another goal was to increase the clients' cueing skills when acting as facilitators during treatment sessions. This was measured by
recording the number of cues that facilitated the partner's recall of
key elements without the assistance of the clinician (which was calculated as a percentage). It was also measured by recording the number of different cueing styles used for each story (e.g., gesture,
writing, providing the first sound of the word).

Qualitative Goals

The following qualitative goals were set for JG and LF:

End-of-Treatment Questionnaire

Client's name: _____

Part A: Program Evaluation

1. What did you enjoy most about cooperative group treatment?

2. What did you find to be most challenging about the program?

3. Overall, do you think the program was worth the time, effort, and cost involved?

    Yes _____ No _____

4. What could we change to make the program more effective for future clients?

Part B: Evaluation of Personal Gains

1. In what ways do you think the treatment program helped you improve your communication skills?

2. Do you feel any different about yourself now as a communicator? If so, please explain.

3. Please list any new responsibilities you have assumed at home or elsewhere since beginning the program.

4. Please list any new hobbies, activities, or relationships you have become involved in.

Thank you for taking the time to provide us with this information.

Figure 2-2. End-of-treatment questionnaire used to gather social validation data for treatment outcome evaluation.

1. Increased dependence on each other and decreased dependence on the clinician were goals for both clients. Progress toward meeting these goals was documented by recording cueing trends at the bottom of the score sheets (see Figure 2-1).

2. Increased awareness of improvements in communication skills during the course of treatment was also a goal for both clients. The clients' daily journal entries were used to assess progress toward meeting this goal.

3. Increased self-confidence as a communicator was established as a goal for both clients. Journal entries, responses to social validation questions (see Table 2-1), and responses to the end-of-treatment questionnaire (see Figure 2-2) were used to document progress toward meeting this goal.

Treatment

When assessment and establishment of goals were complete, the next 14 sessions were scheduled for treatment. Stories for these sessions were selected and presented according to the following order-of-difficulty progression: (1) relatively easy stories were used during the first few sessions, (2) more challenging story tasks were used during the middle stages of the program, and (3) easier story recall tasks were used during the final sessions of therapy. This progression applies the traditional approach for individual treatment sessions—begin with familiar, easy tasks, progress to more difficult tasks, and end with tasks that promote success—to the overall treatment program. This helped desensitize the clients to performance inadequacies in the initial stages of treatment as they were forming a relationship. It also allowed the clients to end the treatment program at the level at which they started, helping them realize the improvement they had achieved.

Four stages of treatment followed the initial assessment sessions. Stage one involved orientation to the therapy approach, using relatively easy procedural story tasks. In stage two, the clients were introduced to more challenging narrative stories. During stage three, the clients completed the most challenging and difficult narrative story tasks. In stage four, the clients returned to easier procedural stories and repeated some earlier narrative tasks. They also practiced improving their discourse skills while recalling personal stories about their future

Table 2-2. Treatment Stages

Stage	Treatment Session #	Difficulty Level	Story Tasks
One	1–3	Easy	Personal introduction stories, procedural stories
Two	4–7	Moderate	Narrative stories, procedural stories
Three	8–10	Difficult	Most challenging narrative stories, procedural stories
Four	11–14	Moderate-to-Easy	Repeated narrative stories, procedural stories, personal narrative stories

plans and societal roles. The four stages of treatment are summarized in Table 2-2. Examples of procedural and narrative stories used during the program are included in Appendix 2B.

Stage One: Orientation to Cooperative Group Treatment (Sessions 1–3)

The first treatment session in stage one involved introducing the clients to one another and discussing the cooperative group treatment approach (see Chapter 1). First, roles were discussed. The clients were presented with a handout (Figure 2-3) that briefly summarized the roles the recaller, facilitator, and clinician would play in large, easy-to-read type. They were informed that their roles would alternate between recaller and facilitator for each successive story.

The clients and clinician then discussed the following treatment sequence:

1. *Presentation of story.* The clinician reads the target story. Some stories (e.g., newspaper articles) are accompanied by pictures, which can be viewed while listening to the story.

2. *Listing of key elements.* The clients work together to compile a list of ten key elements (words or phrases) related to the story. After agreeing on the ten key elements, they record them on a "Key Elements" sheet (Figure 2-4).

Roles in Cooperative Group Treatment

Recaller: Practices retelling a story

Facilitator: Provides the recaller with
cues that help him or her recall all
ten key elements associated
with the story

Clinician: Provides the facilitator with
a cue sheet and suggestions for
cueing, when needed

Figure 2-3. Large-print handout used to describe the roles of the recaller, facilitator, and clinician in cooperative group treatment.

Key Elements

Story: _____

1.
2.
3.
4.
5.
6.
7.
8.
9.
10.

Figure 2-4. Key elements sheet used for recording ten words or phrases that the clients agree are essential to the story.

3. *Cued recall.* The designated recaller practices retelling the story. When the recaller gets stuck (either cannot think of any more key elements or experiences word-finding difficulties recalling a particular key element), the designated facilitator provides cues until all key elements are recalled. Cues can be written, verbal, or gestural. The clinician provides the facilitator with a list of cueing strategies and encourages the use of a variety of cues. The clinician also encourages the recaller to request help when needed.

4. *Recall probe.* The recaller retells the story in 1 minute without cueing assistance from either the facilitator or clinician. The clinician times the recaller with a stopwatch.

5. *Feedback (debrief).* The facilitator provides feedback to the recaller regarding performance during the recall probe. The recaller provides feedback to the facilitator about the effectiveness of cueing skills during cued recall. The clinician provides feedback to both the recaller and the facilitator.

After this orientation, the clients practiced using the treatment sequence for the personal story topic *Introductions.* Each listed ten key elements they thought would be important or interesting when introducing himself or herself to the other. They then took turns following the treatment sequence, alternating as facilitator and recaller. For example, JG showed LF his list of ten key elements. He asked her opinion about whether she thought anything important had been omitted. After the two agreed on his list, he practiced introducing himself to LF, while she held the list. LF provided JG with cues for the key elements he had omitted (e.g., she said "You have five of these" for the key element *five grandchildren* and wrote a number to cue the number of years he had been married). Next, the clinician timed JG with a stopwatch as he introduced himself to LF in 1 minute using all ten key elements. Finally, JG, LF, and the clinician discussed JG's performance during timed recall and LF's performance as the facilitator. Discussion focused on which cues were most helpful, which cueing strategies were not helpful, and what could be done next time to improve performance. LF then proceeded through the same treatment sequence for her introduction. This task was relatively easy for the clients and allowed them to practice the therapy the first time without the stress of remembering the details of an unfamiliar story. It also

---

February 18, 1996
1. Exercised for 45 minutes at the gym.
2. Played my first nine holes of golf with my son since the stroke.
3. Baby-sat the grandkids this evening.

Figure 2-5. Example from JG's daily journal.

allowed the clients to get to know one another better and facilitated discussion between clients and spouses after the session.

At the end of the first treatment session, the clients were provided with journals and informed of their daily assignment: to record three personal events, observations, or activities each day. They were told they would be sharing highlights from these journals with the clinician and each other at the beginning of each subsequent session. An example of a journal entry is included in Figure 2-5.

In the next two sessions of stage one, procedural stories were introduced. At the beginning of each session, the clients shared highlights from their journals. (Topics from these journals were often used by the clinician to create stories for later sessions.) Then a procedural story was verbally presented by the clinician. After this, the clients discussed what they thought were key elements of the story, then they compiled a key-elements list together. An example of key elements selected by the clients for the procedural story *Buying Gas for a Car* is shown in Figure 2-6. Examples of other procedural stories used in cooperative group treatment are included in Appendix 2B.

After selection of key elements, the clients completed cued-recall activities. The recaller then completed the recall probe. From the beginning, emphasis was placed on improving the clients' cueing skills. During the first few sessions, the clients used only a few familiar cueing styles when acting as the facilitator, such as verbally providing the first sound of a word or describing the word. The clients also tended to wait silently for help, rather than requesting help from their partner, when they could not recall a key item. To address this, the clients were provided with lists of strategies they could use. The facilitator's list included "ask a question," "write a few letters," "write the whole word," "describe the word," "say the first sound," "say a rhyme," "spell the word," "write the first letter," "gesture," "use the word in a sentence," "fill in the blank (e.g., say 'pump the _____' for the key element *gas*)," and "draw a picture." The

Buying Gas for a Car

One fact of driving a car is that it runs on gas. When the gas gauge says *empty*, it's time to buy gas. The first step is to find a gas station. Once you find a gas station, you should decide what type of gas you want to buy. Your choices include regular, which is the cheapest; extra, which is slightly more expensive; and supreme, which is the most expensive. As you pull up to the gas pump, you have to remember which side of the car your the gas tank is on, so the gas pump will reach your car. In many places today, you must pay for the gas before you pump it. After you pay for the gas, you can put it in your car. To put gas in your car, you have to take the cap off of the tank. Next, place the gas pump in the tank of your car and fill it up. When the tank is full, the gas pump will automatically turn off. The gas pump should be replaced. Next, you should put the cap back on your gas tank. Following capping your gas tank, you should get your change. Now, you can continue driving to your destination!

1. Empty tank
2. Find station
3. Regular
4. Left side
5. Credit card
6. Pump gas
7. Shuts off when full
8. Hang hose up
9. Cap back on
10. Drive on

Figure 2-6. Procedural story, *Buying Gas for a Car*, followed by key elements selected by JG and LF.

recaller's list included "say you need help," "ask for an opinion," "ask for clarification," and "tell what is and is not helpful." These lists were printed on a sheet of paper as shown in Figure 2-7. The paper was then folded in half along the dotted line and made into a "tent" that could be turned back and forth as the clients switched roles for the stories that were presented in each session. (Two stories were typically completed during each 1-hour session.)

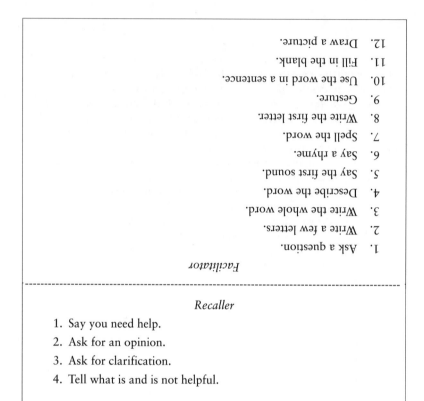

Facilitator

1. Ask a question.
2. Write a few letters.
3. Write the whole word.
4. Describe the word.
5. Say the first sound.
6. Say a rhyme.
7. Spell the word.
8. Write the first letter.
9. Gesture.
10. Use the word in a sentence.
11. Fill in the blank.
12. Draw a picture.

Recaller

1. Say you need help.
2. Ask for an opinion.
3. Ask for clarification.
4. Tell what is and is not helpful.

Figure 2-7. Lists of strategies for the facilitator and recaller to use during cued recall. The form is designed to be folded in the middle along the dotted line and placed on the table as a tent with the appropriate list of strategies facing the appropriate client.

Stage Two: Introduction of Narrative Stories (Sessions 4–7)

Now that the clients were familiar with the steps involved in the therapy, more challenging, narrative stories were introduced and alternated with procedural stories. These included stories about animals (which were accompanied by pictures), similar to *Nile Crocodile*, and newspaper articles of interest to both clients (which were also accompanied by pictures). Some narrative stories were created from information contained in the clients' journals about travel destinations to Alaska and Hawaii. Sometimes, available story materials were greater than 200–250 words in length. In these cases, the clinician reduced the story size. Newspaper articles were successfully shortened to approximately 250 words without eliminating essential information. Examples of narrative stories that were used in therapy are included in Appendix 2B.

During stage two, the clients continued to share information from their journals, began to demonstrate improvement in cueing abilities, and began to depend on each other increasingly for assistance.

Stage Three: Completion of the Most Challenging Story Tasks (Sessions 8–10)

The clients completed their most difficult story tasks during stage three. These were newspaper articles unaccompanied by pictures. In general, these articles were less entertaining and contained more complex and detailed information than those used in stage two. The clinician provided the clients with a variety of newspaper articles. The clients were also encouraged to bring articles from home. The clients then selected the articles they felt contained the kind of important information they would want to relay to their spouse or a friend (e.g., one article they selected reported new research findings on high-fiber diets). For each of these difficult stories, additional time was required to compile the list of ten key elements. The clients were encouraged to review the list to reword phrases that were vague or to eliminate items that were too detailed in nature. Also, because of the increased level of difficulty, the clients had to rely more heavily on their partner for assistance during cued recall. Each client rose to the challenge by increasing creativity in cueing. An increase was also noted in each recaller's requests for assistance. By the end of stage three, the clients were relying on one another far more than the clinician and were providing each other with feedback throughout the treatment sequence not just at its conclusion. Frequent exclamations, such as "You've almost got it!" and "That was a great cue!" were heard.

Stage Four: Transition Back to Easier Tasks and Functional Discourse (Sessions 11–13)

In stage four, the clients returned to procedural story tasks, repeated some narrative stories used in stage two, and practiced improving discourse skills by retelling personal stories about their grandchildren and plans for the future, which was similar to the *Introductions* story task of stage one. Both clients reported that they noticed improvement in the amount of information they were able to recall for both procedural and narrative stories. They also reported increased self-confidence during these sessions. A summary of all stories used in treatment is included in Table 2-3.

Discharge (Session 14)

In addition to completing story recall tasks, discharge activities took place during the clients' final session. These consisted of collecting social validation data, presenting treatment outcome data, and providing a home program. Social validation data were collected using an end-of-treatment questionnaire (see Figure 2-2) and by talking openly with the clients and their spouses about improvements in communication skills and self-esteem they thought were attributable to cooperative group treatment. Treatment outcome data (i.e., percentage scores on recall probes, CIU scores on generalization probes, percentages for successful cueing, and total number of different cueing styles used for each session) were presented in written form to both clients, allowing them to see their improvement from the beginning to the end of the 2-month period.

A home program, included in Appendix 2C, was provided to encourage maintenance of learned skills using the spouses as the communication partners. Although this home program refers to stories used specifically for JG and LF, it could be adapted to accommodate any stories used in a cooperative group treatment program. The following preparation was necessary to create the home program:

- Activity 1. Four familiar procedural stories were selected and tape recorded. A score sheet was created for each story using the

Table 2-3. Summary of all stories used in treatment

Session #	JG	LF
1	PN Personal Introduction	PN Personal Introduction
2	P Planting a Garden	P Going on a Picnic
		P Going out to Dinner (based on personal journal)
3	P Coming to Therapy (based on personal journal)	N Elephant (with picture)
4	N Rattlesnake (with picture) P Going on a Picnic	P Planting a Garden
5	N Blue Bag Bandit (newspaper, with picture)	N Dog Story (newspaper, with picture)
6	N Alaska: The Last Frontier	N Hawaii: The Aloha State
7	P Taking a Trip to Alaska	P Taking a Trip to Hawaii
8	N Flooding (newspaper—*difficult*)	N High Fiber (newspaper—*difficult*)
9	N American Bison (with picture)	N Monarch Butterfly (with picture)
10	P Building a Fire	P Renting a Movie
11	PN Grandchildren (from personal journal)	PN Grandchildren (from personal journal) P Buying Gas for a Car
12	P Buying Gas for a Car	N Hawaii (*repeat*)
13	N Alaska (*repeat*) PN Future (from personal journal)	PN Future (from personal journal)
14	N Exercise	N Exercise

N = narrative story; P = procedural story; PN = personal narrative story (contains personal information).

ten key elements agreed on by the clients (an example is included as Figure 2-8).

• Activity 2. Three familiar narrative stories (with pictures) were selected. Next, the ten key elements the clients selected for each story were printed individually on index cards. A cueing methods sheet was then created for the facilitator, listing the 12 cueing strategies included in Figure 2-7.

• Activity 3. Copies were made of the "Key Elements" sheet (see Figure 2-4) and cueing methods sheet developed for Activity 2.

Example of a Typical Session

The following example describes a session early in stage four of therapy. By this time, JG and LF were beginning to feel comfortable with one another and the therapy, as shown by an increase in their experimentation with cueing strategies and their expressions of humor during the sessions. At the beginning of the session, JG and LF shared personal highlights from their journals. They congratulated each other on the new accomplishments they reported, such as JG's notation that he had played golf for the first time since his stroke. During this session, the clients worked on a narrative story about Hawaii. LF acted as recaller, while JG acted as facilitator. After the clinician read the story to the clients, they discussed the elements they thought were essential. During this time, the clinician provided them with a map of the United States and a copy of the story for reference. After considerable discussion in which they debated which key elements to include and then reworded the phrases until they were as simple and clear as possible, JG and LF chose the following ten key elements: youngest state, Hawaii, Oahu, Maui, Kauai, reached by ship or plane, blue sky and water, beautiful flowers, luau, and hula. Next was cued recall. During cued recall, LF became stuck after talking about Hawaii, Kauai, the blue sky and water, the beautiful flowers, and luaus. After a long pause, the clinician encouraged her to ask her partner for help. LF then told her partner she knew there were more islands on their list, but she could not think of their names. JG successfully cued her by mouthing the letter o for Oahu and verbalizing the first sound in Maui. He then stood up and swayed his body back and forth to cue *hula*. Many cues were required for LF to recall *youngest state* and *reached by ship or plane*.

Home Program

Key Elements and Score Sheet

Story 1: Planting A Garden

Key Element	Recall 1	Recall 2	Recall 3	Recall 4	Recall 5	Recall 6
1. Pick a spot						
2. Sunny and warm						
3. Water supply						
4. Good soil						
5. Select plants						
6. Flowers						
7. Fruit						
8. Vegetables						
9. Get tools						
10. Put plant in hole						
Total correct						

Figure 2-8. Example of key elements and score sheet used for the home program. The ten key elements selected by the partners are listed on the left. The columns to the right provide a space for the clients to score their performance for up to six recall trials for activity 1 (see Appendix 2C). Additional columns could be added, if needed.

The clinician directed JG to his list of cueing strategies and encouraged him to try some different cueing methods. JG experimented with spelling the first word in the phrase, using new gestures, verbalizing the first syllable, and, finally, using description (e.g., saying "it's about how to travel" for *reached by ship or plane*) to facilitate LF's recall of these key elements. Next was the recall probe. LF was able to recall nine of the ten key elements while telling the Hawaii story in 1 minute without cueing. Finally, LF and JG discussed their performance. JG praised LF for getting nine key elements during the recall probe. LF told JG her success was due largely to his cueing. She said the vision of JG dancing the hula made it easy for her to remember to include *hula* in her story. The clients then switched roles with JG as recaller and LF as facilitator for another story task. Increased camaraderie of the clients was evident as the session closed. JG and LF lingered a few minutes to talk with each other about their word-finding problems and the strategies they use in their everyday lives to compensate. It was evident they had learned to rely on each other's opinion and had formed the bond essential to the success of this therapy.

Case Example

LF, a 63-year-old woman, had a left posterior cerebral artery aneurysm and subarachnoid hemorrhage followed by a left frontal craniotomy approximately 1 year before the treatment program. She received speech-language therapy as a hospital inpatient then continued in outpatient treatment for 6 months. After discharge, she pursued therapy at a university clinic. At the beginning of the program, LF reported that she remained troubled by deficits in her communication skills. She appeared anxious regarding her performance during testing and frequently expressed frustration with her word-finding difficulties. LF obtained an Aphasia Quotient of 91.3 on the WAB and scored 36 out of 60 on the Boston Naming Test. Baseline scores for generalization probe stories were 50% CIU per minute for story 1 (*Making Mashed Potatoes*), 41% CIU per minute for story 2 (*Going Fishing*), and 44% CIU per minute for story 3 (*Nile Crocodile*). Results of the American Speech-Language Hearing Association Functional Assessment of Communication Skills for Adults indicated that LF possessed independent communication skills for basic needs and required only minimal assistance from her communication partner in social contexts.

When LF first met JG, she appeared restrained. When learning how to work together to select key elements for a story, LF typically asked JG what he thought and seldom offered her opinion. During initial sessions, LF was able to name key elements with 40–60% accuracy for procedural stories and with 30–40% accuracy for narrative stories. She was able to cue her partner with 50% accuracy during cued recall, using three cueing styles (i.e., providing the first sound, describing the key item, and asking a question). As therapy progressed, LF began to see that her cueing helped JG improve his recall skills. She also observed improvements in her story-retelling skills. Her self-esteem began to grow. She became less restrained and began to participate equally in all components of therapy. She appeared to enjoy getting to know her partner and talking over common problems they shared related to their strokes. LF's recall of procedural stories and narrative stories improved to an average of 65% and 55%, respectively, and cueing skills improved to 80% accuracy. LF was using five cueing strategies, including writing and the use of creative gestures. Scores for generalization probe stories, after four treatment sessions, increased from 50% to 52%, 41% to 43%, and 44% to 49% CIU per minute for stories 1, 2, and 3, respectively.

By stage three of therapy, LF came to sessions eager to share her journal entries. She reported two new activities in her life since starting the program: going out to dinner with friends and beginning a physical therapy treatment program to improve her hand, arm, and leg motor skills. About this time, LF's husband began reporting changes at home. He stated that he thought LF was becoming a more spontaneous and effective communicator, saying he had observed her jump into conversations with friends. He also stated that she seemed much more at ease when conversing over the phone. He reported that she had recently carried on a phone conversation with staff at the Social Security Administration with confidence, a task she would never even have attempted before the treatment program. During this stage the most challenging narrative stories were introduced, and LF's scores dropped back to 40% accuracy; however, at the same time her recall for procedural stories improved to 80–100%. She also achieved 100% accuracy cueing her partner during cued recall, effectively using up to seven different cueing strategies. Scores for generalization probe stories continued to demonstrate improvement, reaching 64%, 55%, and 54% CIU per minute for stories 1, 2, and 3, respectively.

During stage four, LF achieved 90% accuracy for narrative stories. She also maintained skills achieved during stage three for procedural stories and cueing skills. Her post-treatment generalization probe showed improvement over her baseline performance. Her scores improved from 50% to 72%, 41% to 56%, and 44% to 76% CIU per minute for stories 1, 2, and 3, respectively. During her final session, LF expressed pride and pleasure in her progress. Results of her end-of-treatment questionnaire revealed that teamwork and the sense that she was helping her partner were the most enjoyable aspects of therapy and that work on narrative stories was the least enjoyable and most challenging component. She attributed improvements in her communication skills directly to the program, stating that she felt more confident and at ease when talking with friends and strangers. Finally, she emphasized the worth of the program by requesting enrollment in advanced cooperative group treatment.

Important Points About This Treatment

The most notable point about cooperative group treatment is its apparent impact on clients' functional communication skills. In the treatment program described, both clients responded positively to the treatment and improved their story recall and cueing skills. However, in addition to achieving their quantifiable goals and objectives, both clients also reported that they felt new self-confidence as a communicator and that they had resumed certain social activities for the first time since their strokes.

Common Questions and Solutions

Other points surfaced in the form of questions and challenges during the course of treatment. These are presented in the order that they appeared during the described program.

Question: What should the clinician do when the client seems distracted by the stopwatch during the recall probe?

Answer: Be discreet. Stop your scoring at the end of the minute but give the client additional time for recall, if desired. Clients differ. In the program described in this chapter, one client reported the timed aspect of the probe helped recall and one client felt it was distracting.

Question: What kind of stories should be used?

Answer: During the initial assessment sessions, ask the clients about their interests. See what topics they focus on when they first meet one another, then follow their lead. Get ideas from their journals. Encourage the clients to bring in news articles and magazines of interest. You can then rewrite or truncate stories to the desired word length for subsequent sessions.

Question: What if the clients cannot come up with ten key elements?

Answer: Listing fewer than ten key elements is acceptable, depending on the complexity of the story. If fewer than ten key elements are selected, proceed with cued recall until all elements are recalled, then calculate the score for the recall probe as a percentage of total elements recalled.

Question: Who should write down the ten key elements on the "Key Elements" sheet?

Answer: Ideally, clients should alternate the task of recording key elements. However, the member of our dyad who wrote with his dominant hand tended to act as scribe most often. This was due largely to the limited time we had to accomplish all our work each session. More important than recording key elements is agreeing on key elements. While it is not particularly important who writes down the key elements, it is essential that both clients participate equally in the negotiation process.

Question: How does the clinician manage client fatigue?

Answer: Encourage the clients to schedule physically demanding activities after the therapy session. Client fatigue can significantly reduce interaction within the dyad, as well as performance on recall probes. The effects of fatigue on language-task performance has been discussed by Duffy,[5] who summarized that treatment should be conducted in a "success-producing milieu and at a time when the client's physical status during the treatment day is optimal." One of the clients in our dyad attended physical therapy just before each midweek session and demonstrated considerable fatigue and overall frustration on those days. His problem resolved when he changed his schedule.

Question: How does the clinician know how much cueing to provide?

Answer: There is no formula for this, other than to do what is essential to maintain the momentum of the therapy. Each time a long pause occurs during cued recall, it is appropriate to encourage the facilitator to scan the list of key elements for those not yet mentioned and to provide a cue. It is also appropriate to encourage the recaller to ask the facilitator for help.

Question: What should the clinician do if the facilitator uses only a few cueing styles, such as gesture or providing the first sound of a word?

Answer: Provide the facilitator with a list of various strategies, such as those mentioned in Figure 2-7. You may need to model a particular cue so that the facilitator can see its effectiveness. Also, encourage your clients to add their own ideas to the list of strategies. One client in our dyad employed negation in cueing. His humorous cue, "It's not a hot dog stand!" for the key element *gourmet restaurant* helped his partner immediately recall the element and helped her remember to include it again during her recall probe.

Recommended Sources for Materials

An appealing aspect of this treatment approach is that just about anything that interests the clients can be used to develop a story. Procedural stories were developed easily from common knowledge about the steps involved in certain activities (e.g., planting a garden). Narrative stories were composed using readily available reference materials as a guide (e.g., an encyclopedia was used to develop stories about Alaska and Hawaii).

The following is a list of other materials that were used or could be used in cooperative group treatment:

- Clients' journals

- Newspapers

- Magazine articles

- Printouts of news stories or other information accessed through the Internet

- Picture calendars with write-ups on animals, hobbies, locations, or any other topic of interest

- Travel agency brochures

- Maps and atlases (clients can look at these while listening to a location-based story, then the facilitator can use the map or atlas to provide visual cues for key elements during cued recall)

- Children's books (particularly those with a topic focus, such as ocean life or national parks, that contain junior high–level text)

- Cookbooks or any other instructional books (for procedural stories)

References

1. Kertesz A. Western Aphasia Battery. New York: Grune & Stratton, 1982.
2. Goodglass H, Kaplan E. The Assessment of Aphasia and Related Disorders. Philadelphia: Lea & Febiger, 1983.
3. Frattali CM, Thompson CK, Holland AL, et al. American Speech-Language Hearing Association Functional Assessment of Communication Skills for Adults. Rockville, MD: ASHA, 1995.
4. Nicholas L, Brookshire RH. Quantifying connected speech of adults with aphasia. J Speech Hear Res 1993;36:338.
5. Duffy JR. Schuell's Stimulation Approach to Rehabilitation. In R Chapey (ed), Language Intervention Strategies in Adult Aphasia (3rd ed). Baltimore: Williams & Wilkins, 1994;146.

Appendix 2A:
Generalization Probe Stories

Making Mashed Potatoes (Procedural)

Nothing goes better with a pan of gravy than mashed potatoes. However, making mashed potatoes takes many steps. First, you must wash and scrub the potatoes. Once the potatoes are clean, you should use a vegetable peeler or knife and peel the potatoes. When the potatoes are peeled, you should place them in a pot, fill the pot with water, and add a little salt. The pot should be placed on the stove. Bring the water to a boil and cook the potatoes until they are tender. The potatoes are tender when a fork or knife can be inserted in each one easily. When the potatoes are cooked, you will next drain the potatoes in a colander. While the potatoes are still warm, add butter and milk to the potatoes and mix them all together. Some people prefer to use a potato masher for this job, but others prefer to use an electric mixer. After the potatoes, butter, and milk are mixed together into the desired consistency, add salt and pepper to taste. When the mashed potatoes are seasoned like you like them, it's time to serve them.

Going Fishing (Procedural)

A relaxing hobby for many people is going fishing. It takes some skill and quite a bit of good luck. Before going fishing, your first task is to decide what type of fish you would like to catch. Once you decide on the type of fishing you would like to do, it's time to get your equipment ready. Your next job, then, is to select the appropriate fishing rod and reel for fishing. The line must be the right weight for catching the fish. In addition to the rod and reel and the fishing line, you must select the right hook. Next, you have to buy the best bait for the fish. Different fish like different bait. Some popular baits include shrimp, liver, worms, and good old bread. Once you have the bait, it's time to drive or walk to your favorite fishing spot. When you arrive, unload your rod and reel and the bait. Next, bait your hook. Once baited, it's time to cast your line in the water. With a little patience and luck, you'll get a strike soon!

Nile Crocodile (Narrative)

In spite of its name, the Nile crocodile does not live only in the Nile river area. It can be found in many African streams and on the island of Madagascar. The Nile crocodile is hunted for its skin and is an endangered species in several regions. However, it thrives in great numbers in east Africa.

The Nile crocodile spends a great part of its life on sandy riverbanks, warming itself in the sun. Just like a dog, it keeps its mouth open to control its body heat, and it warms its blood from the heat of the sun's rays. And while it keeps its mouth open, it can have some light dental work done. Little birds, called plovers, clean the crocodile's teeth by eating any food trapped between them. This large reptile waits for hours in complete stillness for its prey. When it thinks that its victim is close enough, it springs upon it with astonishing speed. It then drowns its prey in the water and eats it. The Nile crocodile feeds on fish, turtles, birds, and mammals. It can be aggressive toward people who get too close, but most people are careful not to do so.

Appendix 2B: Procedural Stories and Narrative Stories

Procedural Stories

Going on a Picnic

A warm sunny day is an ideal time to go on a picnic. If you decide to go on a picnic, there are various things to do to organize the trip. First, you should pick a place to have your picnic. Favorite picnic spots include the beach, a nearby park, or any place with a special view. With your picnic destination selected, you should decide what time you would like to have your picnic. A lunchtime picnic seems very popular. Next, you should decide what food to take. Some people take what's available in their kitchen, such as a loaf of bread, lunch meat, fruit, and a drink. Others like to prepare a more elaborate meal with fried chicken, potato salad, homemade cookies, and perhaps wine. When your food is ready, it's time to pack it in a picnic basket. Once the food is packed, it's time to drive or walk to your picnic site. When you get to the picnic site, you should claim a picnic table or spread a blanket on the ground. Next, unpack your food. Finally, you can eat and enjoy being outdoors!

Planting a Garden

When planting a garden, there are various steps to follow. First, a spot in the yard must be selected. This spot should have good soil, get plenty of sun, and have a supply of water nearby. Next, you should decide what type of plants you want in your garden. They can include flowers, such as roses, irises, or azaleas. Or, you could pick vegetables, such as corn, peas, or squash. Maybe you would prefer fruits such as watermelon, strawberries, or cantaloupes. Some gardens even have a combination of flowers, fruits, and vegetables! Once the plants have been purchased, you should read the directions attached to the plant. These directions tell how to plant and care for your plant. Next, you have to decide where to put each plant. Once you have decided where to place each plant, a shovel or spade should be used to dig a hole. After placing each plant in a hole, cover the roots with dirt. Once each plant is planted, water thoroughly. The last thing to do is to watch your plants grow!

Renting a Movie

Every now and then, it's fun to rent a movie for some entertainment at home. If you plan to watch the movie with a friend or your wife or husband, the first thing to do is talk about which movie you want to see. You might want to rent an old favorite, like *Casablanca*, or an adventure, like *Crimson Tide*. Or you may be in the mood to see a comedy, like *Grumpy Old Men*. Once you have decided on the movie you want to see, it's time to drive to the video store.

When you get to the video store, the first thing to do is to look on the shelf to find the movie you want. Once you have the movie you want to rent, you must go to the cashier and pay the rental fee. Most rental fees are around 3 dollars. When you pay your rental fee, some video stores ask to see your identification card. That way they can look you up on their computer to see if you owe them any late charges on other movies you have rented.

When you get home from the video store, the next thing to do is to choose what you want to eat while you watch your movie. Some people like to order pizza. Others prefer popcorn and soda. When your food is ready, it's time to put on comfortable clothes, dim the lights, and enjoy the show!

Building a Fire

When the weather gets cold, many people find that a roaring fire is just the thing to take the chill off. Others enjoy the cozy, romantic feeling that a fire adds to any fall or winter evening. However, building a fire can be frustrating for those who have never learned the steps involved.

First, be sure the damper is open. This allows smoke to travel up the chimney rather than pouring into the living room. Next, gather logs, kindling, newspaper, and matches next to the fireplace. Wad single sheets of newspaper into tight balls and place them around the grate. Stack the kindling on top of the newspaper using a grid pattern similar to a tic-tac-toe board. Next, stack three to five logs on top of the kindling. Wood logs should be dry and free of nails, paint, or varnish for them to burn easily and safely. Place the logs at angles to each other. Putting additional wads of newspaper in the crevices created by the logs helps the wood catch on fire.

Finally, use long matches to light many pieces of newspaper. Then, sit back with your cup of hot chocolate and enjoy!

Narrative Stories

Hawaii: The Aloha State

Hawaii is the only state in the United States that does not lie on the mainland of North America. It is made up of a chain of 132 islands located in the middle of the Pacific Ocean. Almost all of the people of Hawaii live on just seven of these islands. Hawaii is the youngest state in the Union, having joined the Union in 1959.

Hawaii is world famous for its beauty and pleasant climate. It has deep-blue seas, brilliantly colored flowers, graceful palm trees, and plunging waterfalls. These attractions provide some of the most thrilling scenery in the United States. Cool Pacific winds keep Hawaii pleasantly mild all year round.

Every year, millions of vacationers travel to Hawaii by ship or by plane. It is one of the favorite year-round playgrounds of the world. Many visitors remain in Honolulu to enjoy Waikiki Beach and other attractions on Oahu. Others prefer the less populated islands. Tourists find excellent hotels on Oahu, Hawaii, Kauai, Maui, and Molokai. Wherever they go, vacationers are likely to attend a luau, featuring delicious Hawaiian food and a dance called the hula. Hula means dancing in Hawaiian. Hula dancers sway their hips and wave their arms gracefully to the rhythm of music. Their movements tell stories and describe the beautiful scenery of the islands.

Alaska: The Last Frontier

Alaska is the largest state in the United States. It is almost one-fifth as large as all the rest of the United States and is more than twice the size of Texas, but Alaska has fewer people than any other state. About 500 miles of Canadian territory separate Alaska from Washington. Because of this, Alaskans often refer to the rest of the continental United States as the "lower 48." The Alaskan mainland's most western point is only 51 miles from Russia. Alaska is the Union's 49th state, having joined the Union in 1959 just before Hawaii.

The name *Alaska* comes from a word used by the people of the Aleutian Islands. The word means great land or mainland. Today, Alaska is often called the *last frontier*, because much of the state is not yet fully settled. Alaska is famous for tall mountains and beautiful scenery. Mount McKinley, which is 20,320 feet above sea level, is the highest peak in the United States. Alaska also has the 13 next highest peaks and almost all of the nation's active volcanoes. Alaska's vast areas of untamed wilderness attract many people who love the outdoors. Expert mountain climbers tackle the highest peaks in North America. Hunters stalk enormous brown bears and swift caribou. People fish for record-sized salmon and trout. Thousands of tourists travel by car, train, boat, or plane each year just to see Alaska's magnificent mountain scenery and historic coastal towns.

Exercise

Exercise is any type of physical activity that uses the muscles of the body. Sports, such as baseball, tennis, and bowling, provide opportunities to exercise, as well as activities like swimming, bike riding, and weight lifting. Even things you do at home such as gardening, painting, and washing floors provide helpful exercise. All of these activities require running, squatting, lifting, or other movements that put the muscles to work.

Exercise is important because it keeps our bodies in good physical condition. It aids health by improving our blood circulation, breathing, digestion, and metabolism, which is the way that our body uses the food we eat. There are psychological benefits to exercise too. Many people sleep better after exercise, wake up more refreshed, and notice improvement in the way they feel during the day.

The American Medical Association offers three important guidelines for anyone who wants to begin a successful exercise program. First, they suggest that you exercise at least three times each week for 20 minutes or more. Second, they say you should start gently, then increase your efforts gradually over the first few weeks. Don't push yourself too hard! Finally, they say you should choose a form of exercise that you enjoy so that improving your health will become a fun and rewarding habit!

Appendix 2C: Home Program

General Instructions

Over the past 2 months, we have worked together in cooperative group treatment to improve communication skills by expanding your ability to recall information and to cue your therapy partner. Throughout all therapy activities, you have demonstrated outstanding motivation and ability to self-monitor your progress. This home program has been created so that you can maintain the progress you have achieved in therapy. All of the activities described below are based on stories or tasks we have worked on throughout the program. I encourage you to work on one of the following activities at least three times each week for at least 20 minutes. Activity 1 requires the use of a tape recorder. All other materials you will need are included with this home program.

Specific Guidelines

Activity 1: Retelling a Story You Hear

This activity is designed to help you practice your story retelling skills for stories that are told in a step-by-step sequence, such as the story *Buying Gas for a Car*. Enclosed with this home program are two cassette tapes. Tape 1 side A contains four stories we worked on in therapy. Tape 2 is a blank tape for you to use to record yourself as you retell each story. Also included are lists of key elements that you and your partner created for each story. These key elements will also serve as score sheets.

1. *Listen.* Listen to the first story on tape 1.

2. *Review.* When the story ends, review the list of key elements for the story.

3. *Retell.* Take out tape 1, insert tape 2, and record yourself as you retell the story without looking at the key elements. As you do this, try to think of cues you and your partner used in therapy that were helpful and try to remember to recall the key elements in the sequence in which they are listed.

4. *Score.* Rewind tape 2 and listen to the story you told. As you do this, check off the key elements you named.

After completing one story, you can reinsert tape 1 and proceed to the next story, or you can rewind the story you just completed on tape 1 and repeat it to see if you can improve your score.

Activity 2: Cueing a Partner

This activity is designed to help you practice your cueing skills. Enclosed with this home program are three animal pictures and the stories about them to use as a reference (e.g., if you forget the significance of a preselected key element, you can refer to the story to clarify it). Attached to each picture are ten key element cards containing individual key elements that you and your partner selected for the animal story. For this activity, you will need a partner, an animal picture with its ten key element cards, and a "Cueing Methods" sheet.

The object of this activity is for one person to hold a key element card and provide cues until the other person (who cannot see the card) correctly names the key element that is written on the card.

1. Place the animal picture on the table where both you and your partner can see it. The first time you practice this activity, you may want to read the story that goes with the picture so that you and your partner will be more familiar with the key elements listed on the cards.

2. Next, shuffle the ten key element cards to ensure they are in random order and place them face down on the table.

3. One person then selects a card without letting the other person see it. That person then uses cueing strategies listed on the "Cueing Methods" sheet or any other strategies he or she can think of until the partner correctly guesses the name of the key element. Try not to write or say the entire name of the key element unless all other cues have been unsuccessful.

4. After the partner correctly guesses the name of the key element, review with that partner the cues that were the most helpful and least helpful.

Activity 3: Retelling a Story You Read

This activity also requires a partner. It is designed to help you practice your story retelling skills for stories that you read in your daily newspaper. For this activity, you need a newspaper and the "Key Elements" and "Cueing Methods" sheets that are included with this home program.

1. *Read.* Select a short newspaper article that interests you, then read it together with your partner.

2. *Record key elements.* Together with your partner, write down ten key elements for the story you read.

3. *Review.* Before retelling the story, review the list of key elements you and your partner created. At this time, you can discuss the story with your partner and the reasons the particular key elements you selected are important.

4. *Retell.* Next, practice retelling the story without looking at the key elements. As you do this, you can have your partner cue you for key elements you do not mention, using any method listed on the "Cueing Methods" sheet.

This activity can be more challenging than activities 1 and 2, because you are working on newspaper stories that we did not practice in therapy. It is not necessary to retell your newspaper stories without cueing, like you did during activity 1, unless you choose to do so to further practice your retelling skills.

Additional Activity: Writing in Your Journal

I also encourage you to continue recording three personal events, activities, or observations each day in your journal. Continued writing practice will help you to maintain and further improve your writing skills and is also a good way to record and remember new activities and accomplishments in your life.

3

Cooperative Group Treatment for Individuals with Mild Head Injury

Laura H. Fisher

This chapter discusses the use of cooperative group treatment with individuals who have sustained traumatic brain injury (TBI). Clinical application of this treatment with two clients, referred to as DG and TC, is the primary basis for the information in this chapter. Because the language and cognitive deficits suffered in TBI differ from those of aphasic clients, appropriate variation of treatment goals and strategies for this population are addressed. Deficits associated with TBI that directly impact the implementation of this treatment include (1) disorganized, tangential discourse; (2) imprecise language; (3) difficulty modifying actions or language; (4) diminished understanding of abstract language; (5) disinhibited or socially inappropriate language; (6) lack of initiation; (7) difficulty comprehending extended spoken or written language, especially under time constraints; (8) difficulty detecting main ideas; (9) a decreased ability to read social or nonverbal cues; and (10) poor deficit awareness.[1] Although the presence of these cognitive-linguistic deficits makes some aspects of this treatment challenging for individuals with TBI, the fact that numerous skills are required to participate in cooperative group treatment is one reason that this is a viable therapy for these individuals.

Determining Which Clients to Group

• *Specific language skills.* Severity level appears to be the most valuable piece of information for determining which clients should be grouped, regardless of the etiology of the brain injury. Severity level can be determined through three baseline measurements of correct information units (CIUs),[2] using 150- to 200-word narrative and procedural stories. An example of appropriate client grouping was the pairing of a 25-year-old female, DG, who was involved in a car accident at age 13, with a 31-year-old man, TC, who had viral encephalitis 3 years before beginning this treatment. They presented with similar baseline measurements in terms of CIUs on the narrative and procedural stories, though the types of errors made were different.

• *Motivation.* Although clients' motivation is a more difficult characteristic to assess, experience indicates that grouping clients with mismatched motivation levels can have a detrimental impact on the therapy process. For example, DG was a motivated client who often appeared frustrated in working with someone who was having more difficulty than herself. Because DG had expressed dissatisfaction when she was previously grouped with someone whose baseline performance was lower than hers, the clinician considered it vital to match her with someone whose language skill severity level was commensurate with, or even slightly higher than, hers.

• *Age.* Age can also be a factor in determining grouping of clients with TBI. In contrast to stroke, individuals with TBI are more likely to be active adolescents or young adults. By grouping clients of similar ages or similar life stages, they are better able to relate to each other in terms of challenges being faced outside of therapy. The grouping of DG and TC was successful, in large part, because they were both single individuals who were trying to reestablish social contacts. Both were also very motivated in their pursuit of careers. Although their interests and personalities were very different, the fact that DG had applied to a physical therapy aide program and TC was trying to maintain his computer business seemed to create a similar sense of purpose in their professional lives.

Psychosocial benefits of group therapy have frequently been discussed in the literature. By grouping partners with similar life challenges, it allows them to brainstorm about solutions to mutual problems and gain insight and support from someone who "has been there." Perceived improvements in self-confidence, interpersonal skills, and coping skills are difficult to measure, though clients and families have reported observing these changes following cooperative group treatment.

- *Interests and personalities.* Matching of interests and personalities appears to be a less valuable indicator of success in grouping clients. In fact, varied interests lead to new learning opportunities for partners. Personality differences can lead to conflicts, especially in clients whose deficits include disinhibited speech or decreased monitoring of their own and their partner's social cues. However, this can create an opportunity to address these deficits in a real-life scenario. Personalities are also difficult to factor into grouping of clients because potential conflicts are both difficult to anticipate before beginning therapy and can dissipate as therapy progresses to the forming stage.

- *Etiology.* The grouping of clients by etiology of brain injury is recommended, as the type of deficits encountered are more likely to be similar. This allows the clinician to focus on related goals for the clients in the group and also reduces the potential for friction between clients. For example, the grouping of TBI and aphasic clients would more likely result in interpersonal conflicts related to disinhibited social behavior than if the group consisted only of clients with aphasia.

- *Other factors.* Criteria not used to group clients include the time after onset, current health status, and education and employment background. Coexisting motor speech diagnoses need only be considered if they result in a significant difference between the clients' efficiency and efficacy of their functional communication skills.

Baseline Assessment and Therapy Outcome Evaluation

- *Western Aphasia Battery.* Expressive and receptive language skills can be measured using the Western Aphasia Battery (WAB).[3] The administration time of the WAB is about 60 minutes.

- *Boston Naming Test.* The Boston Naming Test[4] provides specific information about the clients' degree of word-finding impairments and the effectiveness of different cueing strategies. This information is especially useful in the planning and implementation of treatment. The administration time of the Boston Naming Test is about 15 minutes.

• *American Speech-Language Hearing Associations' Functional Assessment of Communication Skills for Adults.* The American Speech-Language Hearing Associations' Functional Assessment of Communication Skills for Adults (AHSA FACS)[5] indicates the degree of assistance required and the effectiveness and efficiency of communication during functional communication tasks. It is recommended that this be completed after administration of all other aspects of baseline testing. No therapy time is required for administration of this assessment; however, 30 minutes of the clinician's time are required.

• *Clinician-generated probes.* Baseline measurements of narrative and procedural story retelling are instrumental in determining the appropriateness of client grouping. Also, by reviewing written transcripts of baseline story retelling, the clinician gains valuable insight about the types of potential errors that will be encountered in therapy. Baseline measurements are also used to document generalization throughout treatment. Narrative and procedural stories are used as baseline measurements. Generally, procedural stories are easier for clients. One suggestion for selecting baseline stories is to use one procedural story, one narrative story, and a third story that is chosen based on the type of story that will be used most during therapy. The stories used with DG and TC were *Making Mashed Potatoes*, *Going Fishing*, and *Nile Crocodile* (see Chapter 2, Appendix 2A). Each story is presented at least three times to ensure stability of performance. Each story retell is assessed using CIUs.[2]

Procedurally, baseline and probe measures are collected in the following manner. During the two sessions used for assessment, the baseline stories are read by the clinician and recalled by the client both at the beginning and end of the therapy session, for a total of four baseline measures. Although clients are allotted only 1 minute per story retelling, it is suggested that they be allowed to finish the thought or sentence that they are expressing at the end of that time frame. After therapy begins, probe measures are collected once every 2 weeks. Again, the baseline stories are read by the clinician, and the client is allowed 1 minute for verbal recall of the story. The percentage of CIUs to total word count is calculated for each story, and performance is monitored for progress throughout therapy.

• *Social validity.* Social validity measures reflect the effect that clients' communication skills have on their role in the community. At the outset of therapy, clients are asked to set goals for improving their communication. Once every 2 weeks, the clinician initiates a conversation about the clients' perceived progress both in the clinic setting and in everyday situations. At the end of therapy, clients are asked to assess any changes that they feel have occurred in their communication skills. They also set new goals related to their communication interactions outside of therapy, which they are encouraged to pursue with the help of a supportive peer. Examples of social validation questionnaires are in Chapters 2, 4, and 5.

Individual Treatment Measures

After therapy begins, part of the clinician's role is to provide feedback to both the story recaller and the facilitator on their performance. A checklist for each person, written on the same sheet for easy tallying, is suggested. An example of one such form is seen in Figure 3-1. In the first column for the story recaller, the clinician lists the agreed-on key words and phrases. The second and third columns are used during the practice recall phase of the session. The correct and incorrect recall of key words (which are indicated with + and −), without cueing, is indicated in the second column. For those words that are not recalled independently, indicate the type(s) of cue(s) provided by the facilitator and the success of this cue (with a + or −) in prompting accurate recall. The last column, for solo recall, is used to chart the accuracy (with a + or −) of the client's key-word recall during the final 1-minute recall portion of therapy. The lower half of the chart is used only during the practice recall phase of therapy to chart the facilitator's cueing effectiveness, as no cueing is provided during the final 1-minute recall.

Case Example

In the group highlighted in this chapter, both clients scored within normal limits on the Aphasia Quotient portion of the WAB and were able to provide complete written descriptions of the picnic

Story Recaller _____

Key Word	Practice Recall (+ or −)	Type of Cue (+ or −)	Solo Recall (+ or −)
1.			
2.			
3.			
4.			
5.			
6.			
7.			
8.			
9.			
10.			

Percentage correct independently during practice:
_____

Percentage correct independently during solo recall:
_____

Effective types of cues:
_____

Number of requests for help:
_____

Facilitator _____

Key Word	Type of Cue(s) Given	Efficacy (+ or −)
Number of cues provided		
Number of successful cues		
Comments: ability to revise cues		

Figure 3-1. Score sheet used by the clinician for each client's story recall. (+ = client uses the key word or describes the concept represented by the word; − = word or concept not verbalized during recall.)

scene, indicating that they were similarly matched, mildly impaired clients. Both clients also completed nearly all of the functional communication tasks measured in ASHA FACS[5] without assistance, which indicated a mild communication deficit. The greatest degree of breakdown came in the retelling of narrative stories and, to a lesser degree, procedural stories. The primary deficit observed in both clients was a lack of cohesiveness and completeness in the story retelling.

Clinician's Task: Selecting the Goals or Objectives for the Group

The selection of treatment goals is determined through client interviews and analysis of assessment results. In this case study, the clients were performing within normal limits on standardized and descriptive assessment tools. However, it was apparent from client report and clinician-client interaction that clients experienced difficulty in many daily activities, such as taking phone messages accurately and integrating information to discuss or write about work-related topics. They also reported difficulty attaining goals that were important to them, such as meeting new people. The following functional goals were, therefore, selected for these clients:

Quantifiable Goals

1. Increase the cohesiveness and completeness of clients' communicative efficacy in retelling stories, as measured by the total CIUs, total word count, and the ratio between the two.

2. Improve clients' ability to cue their partner or ask for clarification when practicing story retelling, as measured by tracking the number and variety of cues provided or requested and the percentage of effective cues provided.

3. Increase clients' ability to provide and request feedback regarding performance in therapy. This is measured by tallying the quantity of interactions and using a plus or minus (i.e., + or −) evaluation of the effectiveness and appropriateness of these verbal exchanges.

Qualitative Goals

1. Improve clients' functional communication skills, as measured by social validation discussions and checklists.

2. Improve negotiation skills, as observed by the clinician. Qualities evaluated are tactful negotiations, sharing responsibility for choosing key words, and timeliness of key-word negotiations.

Getting Started: Planning Treatment

The challenges of planning treatment include finding and selecting appropriate stories for retelling and deciding what written or visual props can facilitate the clients in their roles of story recaller and facilitator.

Selecting Stories

Sources for stories vary depending on the ability level of the clients. With higher-functioning, young clients, the newspaper is an appropriate source for narrative stories that are current and offer a variety of topics. Because news stories are often lengthy, the clinician should use either the first one-third to one-half of the article or look for brief, eye-catching stories in the travel, sports, or metro news sections.

One of the most entertaining and valuable news stories used in one session was a two-paragraph, 160-word story, brought in by TC, that discussed the opening of a museum of computer relics. On the surface, it appeared to be a dry, overly brief story with little potential. However, the topic was very interesting to TC, and he was able to bring it to life by discussing the meaning and background of many points in the story. Before the retelling of a story, it is sometimes difficult to anticipate what stories will generate good dialogue and debate of key words and provide a valuable language experience. The clinician should look for stories in which there are approximately 20 key words or ideas. Although the clients may not choose any of the key words the clinician anticipated during reading, a story with many logical choices of words will likely yield an appropriate amount of information for clients to build on.

One challenge in scanning news or magazine articles is frequent use of abstract language or inference. Many patients who have suffered dif-

Going bowling is a fun sport to do with a lot of people. When you and your friends get to the bowling alley, the first thing you need to do is decide how many games you plan on playing and pay the cashier for those. The cashier assigns your group a lane and gives you a receipt. Next, you go to the area where you can rent bowling shoes and tell the person working there what size shoes you wear. You can change your shoes at your assigned lane. Then, look for a bowling ball that is a good weight and close fit for your fingers. Someone from the group needs to list the names or initials of all the bowlers on the score sheet so that people can keep track of scores. The score sheet is electronic and can be seen at the desk, in the lane, or up above the lane. Usually, people do one or two warm-up throws before beginning the scoring. Then, you can begin bowling.

Figure 3-2. *Going Bowling*: Procedural story composed by DG and TC.

fuse brain damage have difficulty with abstract language and inference. For that reason, appropriate literature written for middle-school students is a good source of material. Another valuable feature in some newspapers is a daily column for adults learning to read. These news stories are current but are written with more simplistic language and in a more linear fashion than general news articles.

Published versions of procedural stories suitable for conversation are difficult to find. Clients or the clinician can write stories that are pertinent to the interests of the clients. For example, DG and TC put together a brief story about the steps involved in going bowling after they realized they both had experience with this pastime (Figure 3-2).

Written or Visual Cues

The type and quantity of visual cues depend on the abilities of the group members. Even though clients may not appear to need the structure provided by cues or may indicate that they do not need it, it is recommended that visual reminders be provided to clients, at least at the beginning of therapy. For the facilitator, a list of different types of cues can be provided (Table 3-1). For example, the facilitator may "ask a question" or "say the first sound" to cue the story recaller. The story recaller also can benefit from written suggestions that can be used when he or she gets

Table 3-1. Cue Sheet: Written Cues Provided to the Facilitator

1. Ask a question.
2. Gesture or pantomime.
3. Say the first sound of the word.
4. Say the function of the word.
5. Describe the word.
6. Write or spell part of or all of the word.
7. Say the word in a sentence.
8. Draw a picture of the word.

stuck during the retelling. Examples of such suggestions are "visualize the story" and "ask your partner a question" (Table 3-2).

Six-Step Treatment Process

Step One: Getting to Know the Clients (Session 1)

A functional icebreaker for the first session is to have clients brainstorm together about the types of things they would like to learn about people when they first meet them. Obviously, each group's final list of items will be different. For example, DG and TC, both single clients, included age, marital status, occupation, where they live, who they live with, hobbies, and education on their list. Next, the clients should use the list of ten items to discuss their own backgrounds. The clients are then introduced to the cooperative group treatment process by retelling the information they have learned about their partner in 1 minute. Because the topic is inherently interesting to both parties and the type of characteristics being discussed are familiar, the act of retelling and cueing are relatively easy. In a short period of time, the partners have learned a lot of information about each other in a nonthreatening way and have begun to learn about the therapy.

Following introductions, the clinician should explain to the clients how the roles of facilitator and story recaller, which they have just completed, are repeated with different types of stories. Confidence in the process is enhanced by explaining the documented benefits of this therapy.

During the first session, it is crucial to discuss the importance of attendance. Indicate that prompt, regular attendance shows a commitment

Table 3-2. Cue Sheet: Written Cues Provided to the Recaller

---

1. Visualize key words.
2. Say a word(s) that is similar to the key word.
3. Ask a question.
4. Talk out loud about what you can remember.

---

to the partner's, as well as individual, progress. Capable clients should establish a routine of writing in a journal on a daily basis as part of the homework. Writing a paragraph describing three things the client did that day and reading selected entries at the beginning of the following session often creates opportunities for original stories, provides insight to their interests, and is a way of gathering social validity information.

Step Two: Procedural Stories (Sessions 2 and 3)

Procedural stories are recommended early in therapy, because they are less demanding and allow the clients to be successful while they familiarize themselves with the cooperative group treatment process. Examples of stories that were used during the first two to three sessions are *Building a Fire*, *Renting a Movie* (see Appendix 2B), and *Preparing for a Job Interview* (see Appendix 3A). Stories are intended to describe functional activities that clients are familiar with or are interested in learning about. While the clinician reads the story aloud, the clients have a written copy of the story in front of them. Providing only one copy of the story for the group can promote more cooperative interaction during the actual key-word selections, because the clients are required to share the written material.

Key-Word Selection

During the initial sessions, the processes of forming and storming are taking place (see Chapter 1). For this reason, the clinician takes on a greater role in facilitating the selection and negotiation of ten key words from each of the stories at this early stage. For example, if one client appears overly polite or intimidated and is allowing the other client to make the majority of decisions regarding word choices, the clinician should direct the more passive partner to choose the next word. Another suggestion is to ask a question about a key passage to elicit opinions from the group members.

With clients with TBI, the clinician can be challenged by the interpersonal nuances of forming and storming. The deficits among these clients can range dramatically, making it difficult to generalize potential sources of conflict during these two stages. However, reduced affect, the decreased ability to interpret nonverbal speaker cues, and disinhibition can create less-productive client interactions. The clinician can use such situations to teach social interaction skills to the group or can choose to discuss these problems with clients individually. For example, in the first few sessions, DG was often outspoken to the point of being insulting in her critique of TC's selection of key words, which did not agree with her choice of key words. She appeared unaware of the tension this behavior created. The clinician and DG privately discussed ways to resolve differences of opinion.

Story Retelling

The next step in the process is for one client to act as the story recaller. That person practices retelling the story, without seeing the ten key words, while the other client, the facilitator, listens. The facilitator then provides cues regarding missed words either at the end of retelling, when the recaller becomes stuck, or when the recaller asks for assistance.

Several potential problems can occur at this point in the process. For example, TC, whose memory skills were significantly better than his discourse skills, repeatedly listed the ten key words or phrases rather than integrating the words in a story-telling fashion. This, of course, provided a false picture of his degree of accuracy and timeliness in the story recall phase. Other potential problems include a facilitator who appears to withhold cues for competitive reasons, or who uses only one or two types of cues, or who has difficulty revising unsuccessful cues. All of these problems should be discussed during the brief wrap-up that follows the practice story retelling. For example, after discussing these problems, TC and DG decided to refer to the written reminders (see Tables 3-1 and 3-2) more frequently when acting as recaller and facilitator. They also opted to provide more specific feedback to each other about what types of cueing were the most helpful to them during recall.

After the practice story recall, the clinician asks the facilitator to comment on the recaller's performance and vice versa. Frequently, TC and DG began their feedback to each other by saying, for example, "You forgot...." or "You didn't....," and would list each other's errors or weaknesses. Encourage clients to use a 2 to 1 or 3 to 1 ratio of positive comments to constructive criticism. The clinician can directly or indirectly model the delivery of these comments in his or her portion of the wrap up.

During the next step, the story recaller retells the story in 1 minute without assistance. Again, a brief wrap up, first by the facilitator and then by the clinician, follows the retelling. For example, the facilitator comments on the quantity of correct key words provided by recaller. Next, the clinician adds comments related to the cohesiveness of the 1-minute story retelling and provides suggestions as to how to improve any difficulties that the recaller encountered. The goal is to include two stories in a 1-hour session. The clinician should alert the clients to this expectation to help facilitate the steps of therapy.

Step Three: Single-Subject Narrative Stories (Sessions 3 and 4)

During this step, narrative stories were introduced to DG and TC. The initial choices appeared to be too easy for these clients. The stories were approximately 150 words and involved information about a specific subject. For example, one story involved information about the habitat, diet, and routines of the black bear. The facts in these stories were concrete, the primary subject did not change, and the types of facts discussed were logical associations with the subject. This provided a useful transition from procedural stories to more advanced narrative stories, but it was only used for a short time because these stories were not challenging enough for the higher-functioning TBI clients. Perhaps because of their age, the clients also appeared bored with the animal stories that were used in this stage of therapy.

Step Four: Narrative Stories of Increasing Complexity, Length, or Both (Sessions 5–11)

This stage of cooperative group treatment is the most successful, most challenging, and lengthiest segment of the process. During step four, news stories are the primary source of materials used in therapy.

The key elements to consider when determining the appropriateness of news or magazine articles is length, clarity, and content. Suggested length of news stories is 200–300 words. Many longer stories can easily be shortened. If articles exceed 400 words, the key-word selection becomes too time consuming. Stories presented in a linear sequence with few abstract words are easier to follow than stories with implied sequences and meanings. For example, a brief news article about Martin Luther King's life was easy to follow and facilitated key-word selection. A less successful example was an article on the benefits of art therapy. It had significantly fewer facts, relied on abstract language, and had no obvious structure for the order in which the information was presented. The last factor is content. When news articles are used that contain information that the clients relate to or contain stories that are familiar from radio or television, the process is more successful than if the topic is removed from the lives of the clients. It often is helpful to have clients bring in articles of interest. To ensure their appropriateness, the clinician reviews these articles for use in the following session.

By this step in the therapy process, the clients are familiar with their roles at each stage of the session. They take on more responsibility in the session in both the key-word selection and in providing feedback to each other about their effectiveness as a story recaller or facilitator. The clinician is in the unique and enjoyable position of simply facilitating the forward progression of therapy.

Facilitation by the therapist was consistently required for several problems at this phase. For example, TC and DG often took 20–25 minutes to select 10 key words, because of power struggles over their choices. When the process took this long, it only allowed one story to be completed per session. Intervention by the clinician was required not only to speed up the process but also to encourage both clients to be more tactful and cooperative in their key-word choices. Several strategies were attempted, including (1) setting a time limit of 10 or 15 minutes to determine eight to ten key words, (2) asking clients to read the article and pick out their choices of key words before the session, (3) having the clinician ask pointed questions following the story and encouraging clients to use portions of the answers as key words or phrases, and (4) asking the partners to take turns providing the key words.

When lengthy negotiations and discussions over key-word selection are valuable to the clients' progresses, the tradeoff of only doing one story per session is worthwhile. In that case, the clinician should allow the clients to each act as story recaller and facilitator for that session's selected story. The remaining time should be used in the session to have one client recall a story used in a previous session, discuss stories from the homework journals, or ask questions about the article. Another approach to saving time is to say which of the two partners will be the recaller before initiation of the key-word selection process. The facilitator is generally more willing to forfeit opinions if he or she knows that it is not necessary to recall the words. However, this strategy should be used sparingly, as it can decrease the quality and quantity of the language interaction. The key is to be flexible in determining what time requirements lead to the most productive sessions for the individuals in a group.

Step Five: Clients' Stories (Sessions 12 and 13)

The use of clients' stories grew naturally from the homework journals of DG and TC. Discussion of these entries always took place at the beginning of the session. Although many stories seemed interesting, there was little time to ask questions and learn more about these real-life events. If a story piqued the interest of the clinician and the partner, the client was asked to write up a longer version of the story for the next session or verbally communicate the story sequence at that time. This was appealing to DG and TC, as both clients were interested in improving writing skills.

In addition to writing skills, using clients' stories also built on other previously untargeted skills for the participants. The story recaller told his or her partner's original story. Therefore, the recaller had to use effective listening skills during the reading of the partner's story and ask clarifying questions during the key-word selection, as well as recall the events of the story in a conversational manner. The facilitator, who was also the original story writer, had to effectively communicate the key points of the story in writing and verbally during the story reading and key-word selection. As was true with printed stories, the facilitator also had to listen for accuracy of the story line during the story recall.

TC created a narrative story about an accident he came across on his way home late one night. DG created a different narrative story, more of a single-subject narrative, about the muscles of the back. This story coincided with an anatomy and physiology course she was taking. In addition, the clients together wrote a procedural story about going bowling, an activity they had done together (see Figure 3-2).

Step Six: Combination of Steps Four and Five (Sessions 14–17)

At this point in therapy, both the complex narratives and client-generated stories are used. DG and TC reportedly preferred the narrative news articles because they were more challenging; therefore, these became the focus of therapy. However, sharing the journal entries and including several of the expanded entries enhanced social skills between the clients. Since these stories are interesting for the participants, they are recommended as fillers when there is not enough time to complete a more complex story.

Discharge from Therapy

At the completion of cooperative group treatment, the clients' progress with communication skills is discussed. The clinician shows clients the outcome data for the three untrained baseline stories used to measure generalization; notes behavioral changes seen in the clients' discourse skills; and discusses trends observed in the accuracy of key-word recall, changes in story length and complexity, and clients' abilities to facilitate through effective cueing.

As part of social validation measurement, the final journal assignment is to list the changes that the clients feel have occurred over the course of treatment, if any. Also, clients are asked to outline new goals that they would like to accomplish in their everyday life. For DG and TC, the clinician encouraged them to brainstorm about ways they could build functional communication skills through greater involvement in the community, such as through volunteer work, social groups, or adult education. The clients and clinician then brainstormed about ways to accomplish those goals. DG and TC kept informed of each other's progresses on goals for at least 6 months after the official termination of group therapy.

Upon discharge, clients are provided with a home program that supports the goals worked on in cooperative group treatment (Appendix 3C). Because DG and TC were busy, single individuals, activities were designed that could be completed relatively independently. It is recommended that clients complete an activity from the home program at least three times per week to maintain or build their skills.

The three home program activities used for DG and TC consisted of the following:

• Short news articles followed by specific questions that were used to facilitate key-word selection. Clients were to tape record story retelling or work with a partner. The goals of this activity were to improve the ability to determine key ideas and to improve discourse skills.

• Procedural stories in which the sentences comprising the story were scrambled. Clients were to rewrite the story in sequential order, answer specific questions to facilitate key-word selection, and practice retelling the story using a tape recorder or working with a partner. The goals of this activity were to improve the ability to present ideas in a logical order, the ability to determine key ideas, and improve discourse skills.

• Writing paragraph-length narratives or procedural stories using a key-word outline, topic sentence, support sentences, and a closing sentence. The clients were also encouraged to continue writing in their journals. The goals of this activity were to improve writing skills and to improve presentation of ideas in a logical order.

Example of a Typical Session

This session took place about midway through treatment (session 7). As they entered the room, the clients sat facing each other and the clinician sat at the end of the table. After 1–3 minutes of social conversation, the clinician asked for a volunteer to read several homework journal entries. TC read an entry about some strange noises his car was making. DG asked the follow-up question, "What did the mechanic say about your car?" Next, DG read several of her journal entries. The clinician checked completed homework, although only about one-third of it was read aloud. This part of the session lasted for 5–8 minutes.

Next, the clinician read aloud a newspaper article about a store that provides free career clothing for women who have been on welfare and are returning to the work force. The article included a profile of a young woman who used the store's services. DG, the more dominant member of the group, offered several facts about the woman (e.g., the trade school that she attended) as the starting point for key-word selection. TC disagreed, indicating that he thought the first key-word should be taken from the headline. This strategy had been recommended in the past. The clinician kept quiet for the moment.

When TC started to agree with DG's "less ideal" word choice, the clinician intervened by asking, "What is the article about? Is it about this particular woman or about what this store is doing?" DG immediately responded that it is about the woman but finally conceded that that was of lesser importance. As was typical of this group, deciding on the first word took 5 minutes and involved intense debate. Both clients wrote down the first key word on their own piece of notebook paper. TC, adopting the strategy just used by the clinician, asked DG a question about the store's location to elicit a potential second word. DG questioned the importance of including this fact and offered her own word choice. TC complied with her choice. A similar scenario was carried out for the third word, only by this time, TC was not willing to concede his opinion. The clinician reminded them that there were still eight words to be chosen in 10 minutes. The clinician suggested that TC's choice be allowed to stand for the third word, since DG picked the second word. This reminder to work as partners to accomplish the task appeared to improve their cooperative skills and words four, five, and six were chosen relatively quickly.

Next, a decision was made about whether to include information about the woman profiled in the article or elaborate on the types of services provided by the store. The clinician thought the emphasis should be on the latter but allowed the clients to discuss their views without input. This time, they agreed and focused on the woman in the story. The clinician posed several questions such as, "How did she get off welfare?" and "What type of job does she hope to get?" These questions helped DG focus on relevant information instead of less-relevant details (e.g., the name of the school the woman attended). These questions encouraged the clients to work together to find a mutually agreeable answer.

Due to time constraints, the clients were encouraged to each provide one of the last two key words. Even though TC agreed to the timesaver, he questioned the validity of his partner's choice and subsequently was reminded of his agreement. As always, the key-word negotiation led to a great deal of dialogue. Completion of the key-word selection took 20–25 minutes.

The clinician reviewed the list of words selected by the clients and ensured that each person's list contained the same words. Next, DG was informed that she would be the first recaller. She looked over the list of ten words, mouthing them to herself, and then turned over her piece of paper. TC looked at the list of key words and a list of facilitating cues, as DG began talking about the store that helps needy women. After 50 seconds, DG stopped her story recall because she could not think of anything else to say. She had missed one or two words and asked TC to give her a hint. He provided the cue that he inevitably provided first, saying, "the first letter of the word is *d*." DG could not think of the word and asked for another cue. TC said the first syllable of the word, "do," which again was unsuccessful. The clinician suggested that he ask a question that would elicit the word and he asked, "Where does the store get the clothes from?" DG correctly provided the answer "donation."

TC provided feedback to DG about her performance as a recaller. He commented on her 90% accuracy and her speed. DG then provided feedback to TC on his facilitation abilities. She indicated that the first letters of words were difficult cues for her. The clinician commented on the conversational style of DG's story recall and the appropriateness of the question cue provided by TC. Next, DG briefly scanned the ten key words again. The clinician started her stopwatch as DG retold the story. At the end of 1 minute, DG said nine of ten key words. TC complimented DG on her performance.

Case Example

History and Initial Testing

DG, a 25-year-old female, sustained a closed-head injury at 13 years of age as the result of an automobile accident. She remained comatose for 7 weeks. Traditional therapy had previously been provided; goals of this therapy reportedly included functional memory skills and appropriateness of expressive language. When she began participating in cooperative group treatment, she indicated that she did not socialize often and was not very active in the community. In her first group treatment experience, DG worked with a man who was slightly older than herself and moderately impaired. The mismatched severity levels were not especially significant, but DG reportedly became easily frustrated with her partner. Therefore, she came to her second cooperative group treatment assignment with experience in the process and of being the better performer in a pair.

During assessment, DG scored within normal limits on the WAB.[3] On the Boston Naming Test,[4] she spontaneously named 42 of 60 (i.e., 70%) of picture items correctly. Scores on the Social Communication and Communication of Basic Needs subtests of ASHA FACS[5] (6.7 of 7.0 and 6.8 of 7.0, respectively) supported the overall diagnosis of mildly impaired language skills. DG was able to communicate functionally without assistance in nearly all situations.

Behavioral Observations

Initially, DG exhibited a defensive, aloof posture towards TC. She demonstrated this by orienting her body posture to the clinician, directing many comments to the clinician, and directly criticizing TC's contributions. By the beginning of the third week, DG's language was less confrontational when she disagreed with her partner and she did not look to the clinician to support her point of view. Although she was still likely to express harsh opinions, she was more likely to begin a keyword discussion with a question like "What about..?" instead of "No, that's not..." One of the most enjoyable changes observed was DG's increased use of humor, laughter, and sharing of personal stories and goals. Although she was still competitive, she became more likely to admit when she was wrong or confused about a story.

Therapy Outcome Data

DG showed significant improvement in the ratio of CIUs to total word count across all three untrained baseline stories. The greatest improvement was noted in the baseline narrative story; narrative stories were the primary focus in this group's therapy. Specifically, DG showed noticeable improvements in her ability to transition between sentences and use specific language to communicate a story.

For the procedural story *Making Mashed Potatoes*, DG's baseline scores averaged 66.3%. Subsequent scores for this story, taken every 2 weeks, improved to 79%, 74%, and 79%. For the procedural story *Going Fishing*, her baseline scores averaged 71.1%. Subsequent scores for this story improved to 82%, 88%, and 85%. For the narrative story *Nile Crocodile*, DG's baseline scores averaged 67.2%. Subsequent scores for this story improved to 78%, 82%, and 90%.

Social Validation

When she completed this treatment, DG indicated that she felt she had increased her self-confidence and interpersonal skills significantly through this process. Her mother agreed with these observations. Individual therapy was recommended following cooperative group treatment so that DG could work more specifically on pragmatics and abstract language (the two areas that most interfered with her success in cooperative group treatment). Shortly after the completion of cooperative group therapy, DG attained a job as a physical therapy assistant, which was a goal she had been pursuing for 6 months. She therefore chose to discontinue therapy.

Important Points About This Treatment

1. TBI clients have the opportunity to improve social skills, as well as discourse skills, through cooperative group treatment.

2. The use of narrative stories related to current events is interesting to clients and often leads to extended discourse practice, such as discussion of opinions.

3. Journal entries lead to client-generated stories, build writing skills, and increase discourse related to functional topics.

4. Group dynamics require flexibility. The clinician may find it necessary to adjust expectations about the amount of material covered or the types of interactions between clients depending on the rhythms of the group.

5. The clinician should frequently provide examples to clients about how the communication goals and skills being learned in cooperative group treatment relate to the clients' everyday lives.

Common Questions and Solutions

Question

What can I do when clients take a long time to agree on key-word choices?

Possible Solutions

• Set a time limit of 10 or 15 minutes to determine key words.

• Ask clients to read the article and pick out their choices of key words before the session.

• Ask pointed questions after the reading of the story or when clients disagree and have the clients use portions of the answers as key words or phrases.

• Have the partners take turns providing the seven to ten key words.

• Use only one story per session and have both clients act as recaller for that story.

Question

What should the clinician do when client's recall information is correct, but he or she simply lists the key words or presents information out of order during story recall?

Possible Solutions

• Count as accurate only those key words that are used in complete sentences and are presented in a logical sequence.

• Remind clients that the goal is to increase their conversational skills outside of therapy, rather than to test their memory of ten items.

• During feedback, always include comments about the naturalness of the client's discourse.

Question

With TBI clients, what steps should be taken to address inappropriate social behavior?

Possible Solutions

• If more than one client exhibits such behavior, discuss and model alternative ways of interacting with the group. Together, set goals, provide feedback, and monitor progress over time.

• If only one client exhibits poor pragmatic behavior, address this individually outside of therapy. Discuss ramifications of the behavior, model alternative actions, and agree on goals that will be monitored and discussed independently.

Question

What is helpful if one person consistently dominates the direction of key-word selection?

Possible Solutions

• Ask a pointed question to the less-involved person and suggest that that word or phrase be used.

• Comment on the value of the less-involved person's attempts to provide input.

• Because the dominant person may not be aware of this pattern, point out that his or her choices (for example) have been used for the last four key words and that the partner should choose the next key word.

• Choose a story that the less-dominant partner is interested in or knowledgeable about, so that he or she is more comfortable verbalizing opinions.

Question

Does it matter if the client uses a different but related key-word during story recall?

Possible Solution

• Because the goal is to improve discourse skills, recall of the exact key word is not necessary. For example, if the key word is *career* and the recaller says "job" or "what the person does for a living," the response is considered accurate. Also, the key-word list may contain key phrases as well as single words. Using multiple phrases, however, may make it difficult for clients to remember the information.

Recommended Sources For Materials

The following are sources for narrative stories that are appropriate for clients with high-level abilities:

- Tasks of Problem Solving, stories by LinguiSystems (1992).[6] Sample stories are in Appendix 3C.

- Newspaper articles, especially short articles and summaries (e.g., letters to Dear Abby, travel section write-ups, world-news summaries)

- Magazines

- Literature intended for adults learning to read (look at the library and in your local paper)

- Auditory-comprehension materials for middle-school and high-school students

- Current news feature magazines for middle-school and high-school students

- *Spotlight* by Steck-Vaughn Company, *Stars* by Turman Publishing, or *Sports Illustrated for Kids* by Time, which can be found in a teacher's supply store.

- Encyclopedia entries

- Books of short stories

The following are sources of procedural stories that are appropriate for clients with high-level abilities:

- The crafts, handyman, or cooking sections of the Sunday newspaper

- Sequencing materials intended for students

- Stories written by the clients, the clinician, or both

References

1. Frattali CM, Thompson CK, Holland AL, et al. American Speech-Language Hearing Association Functional Assessment of Communication Skills for Adults. Rockville, MD: ASHA, 1995.

2. Goodglass H, Kaplan E. The Assessment of Aphasia and Related Disorders. Philadelphia: Lea & Febiger, 1983.
3. Kertesz A. Western Aphasia Battery. New York: Grune & Stratton, 1982.
4. Nicholas L, Brookshire RH. Quantifying connected speech of adults with aphasia. J Speech Hear Res 1993;36:338.
5. Ylvisaker M, Szekeres SF. Communication Disorders Associated with Closed Head Injury. In R Chapey (ed), Language Intervention Strategies in Adult Aphasia (3rd ed). Baltimore: Williams & Wilkins, 1994;546.
6. Zachman L, Barrett M, Huisingh R, et al. Tasks of Problem Solving: A Real-Life Approach to Thinking and Reasoning. East Moline, IL: LinguiSystems, Inc., 1992.

Appendix 3A:
Procedural Stories

Preparing for a Job Interview

Several people may be right for a job. That's why interview skills are so important. Those skills may be what gets you the job! There are several steps to take in preparing for a job interview.

First, try to learn about the duties of the job. Be able to discuss relevant coursework that you've completed. Also, think about the skills or experiences you have had outside of school that have prepared you to effectively perform those duties.

On the day of the interview, pay special attention to your appearance. Select clothes that are neat, clean, comfortable, and proper. Be on time! Being late for an interview leaves the impression that you may be late for the job, if you are hired.

During the actual interview, remember to speak clearly and confidently. Listen carefully to what the interviewer has to say. When asked a question, be sure that you answer the question but avoid long, tangential responses. Toward the end of the interview, the employer may ask if you have any questions. Ask questions that show your interest in the position, not questions about the amount of vacation time you will receive! As you leave the interview, be sure to thank the interviewer for their time and interest. Follow-up with a phone call or thank-you letter in the next several days.

Appendix 3B:
Home Program (Provided
on Discharge from Therapy)

General Directions

During cooperative group treatment, we have focused on improving your ability to determine the key ideas in narrative and procedural stories, retell these stories using key concepts, and write summary sentences and paragraphs about stories or personal activities. Your home program is intended to give you additional practice in these areas. Every week, I recommend that you practice at least one item from each of the three activities listed below to maintain the excellent progress you have made in therapy. Share the completed activities with your next clinician, obtain feedback about your work from someone supportive and capable, or both.

Specific Instructions

Activity 1: News Stories

1. For each of the five attached news stories, read the story and answer the questions. These questions are designed to help you pick out the main ideas in the stories and summarize the information.

2. Use the answers from the questions to put together lists of eight to ten key words.

3. After you have completed this, practice retelling the story in your own words. It may be helpful for you to record yourself so that you can review how accurately you have told the story, or work with a partner who can give you feedback about the accuracy or completeness of your story retell.

The following are examples of the topics and corresponding questions in the news stories:

Topic: Girls' Versus Boys' Math Scores in a Recent Study

Questions

- What is the main subject of this article?
- How old were the students included in this study?
- What areas of math were tested (e.g., algebra, geometry)?
- Was there any difference in the scores between boys and girls?

Topic: Editorial on Tunnel Detours for Trucks Carrying Hazardous Materials

Questions

- What is the main subject of this article?
- What are the current laws regarding tunnel detours for commercial trucks?
- What is one reason for tunnel detours?
- What is one reason against tunnel detours?
- How does the person writing this article feel about tunnel detours?

Topic: Upset Victory in a Local Congressional Race

Questions

- What is the main subject of this article?
- Who was involved in the race?

• How long had the previous congressman been in office?

• What was different about the types of voters who turned out for this election?

Activity 2: Procedural Stories

1. To express yourself clearly, it is important to present your ideas in a logical order. For each of the five attached procedural stories, the sentences are written out of order. Rewrite the paragraph, putting the sentences in logical order. Use transitional words like *first, second,* or *next* to help make the time sequence clear.

2. Use the answers from the questions to put together lists of eight to ten key words.

3. After you have completed this, practice retelling the story in your own words. It may be helpful for you to record yourself so that you can go back and review how accurately you have told the story, or work with a partner who can give you feedback about the accuracy and completeness of your story retell.

The following is an example of a procedural story, presented out of order, with a series of corresponding questions:

Topic: Putting Baby to Bed

• As you read the story and gently rock in the rocking chair, it is hoped that the baby will become sleepy.

• Good stories might be *Good Dog, Carl,* or *The Cat in the Hat.*

• Run a small amount of warm, sudsy water in the bathtub and put the baby in the tub for a bath.

• It's after dinner and the baby is tired.

• When you finish reading the story, it's time to put the baby in bed.

• The first thing to do is to bathe the baby.

• When the baby is dry, put soft, clean pajamas on the baby.

• As you enter the baby's room, select a book so you can read a favorite bedtime story.

- It's now time to put the baby to bed.

- After a few minutes of splashing, it's time to rinse the baby off.

- Your final job is to tuck the baby in for the night.

- Once the story is selected, it's time to sit in the rocking chair and read the story.

- When all of the soap is rinsed off, grab a towel.

Questions

- What is this story about?

- What is the first step in putting baby to bed?

- Describe the bath water.

- What must be done after you wash the baby and before you dry him or her?

- What does the baby wear to bed?

- Where do you sit to read bedtime stories?

Activity 3: Writing Original Stories and Journal Entries

I.   Think of an activity that you participated in or something that happened to you recently.

   A.   Jot down a list of the key events in the order in which they occurred. These are just notes for you to work from and should be just key words or phrases, rather than sentences. For example:

   Movie *Broken Arrow*

   Friends

   Dinner

   Out of town

   Good reviews

   Action movie

   Disliked plot

B. Write a topic sentence that tells the reader what the paragraph is about. For example: "I need to learn to trust my instincts about whether I am going to enjoy a movie."

C. Write three to six support sentences that tell the sequence of events that happened or the most important elements of the event. For example: "Recently, several friends called my husband and me and asked if we wanted to go see the movie *Broken Arrow* and then go out for dinner. Although I don't normally enjoy action films, we considered going because we were excited to see the friends who had invited us, since they live out of town. Besides, my husband reasoned, the reviews in the newspaper were good, so it couldn't be that bad. I know that a lot of people enjoy films that involve secret military missions, exploding vehicles, and women with perfect make-up and bodies running along the tops of trains. However, I was happy to see the credits appear at the end of the show."

D. Write a closing sentence that tells how the story ends or what you learned from the story or think of the story. For example: "Next time, I'll remember to trust my instincts about a movie and offer to meet everyone for dinner afterwards!"

II. Continue writing two to three sentences per day about things that you do, see, or learn about to maintain your skills in writing summary sentences. The following is an example of a journal entry: "It was a beautiful day today, so I decided to do as much as possible outside. I walked to the grocery store and bought food for dinner. Then, on the way home, I decided to sit in the park and just watch all the kids playing together."

Appendix 3C:
Narrative Stories*

Spinning Yarns More Than Tall Tales

LANCASTER, Pa.—Historians say a renewed interest in our heritage is now reaching many corners of the country, including business communities. Before the Industrial Revolution, most of our country's products were handcrafted by people trained by their elders. These customized products reflected each individual crafter's pride and personality.

Elsie Moore, owner of Spinner's Wheel, is just one of many business founders who has gone back in time to earn her living. Moore spins yarns to sell to weavers who make custom clothing and interior decorations like rugs and wall hangings.

Moore's customers say she spins another kind of yarn, too. Moore is a gifted storyteller who captures the imagination of all who come to her shop to see her handiwork and hear her tales.

"I grew up listening to my grandfather tell stories while sitting on his porch on Sunday afternoons. Some of them were tall tales and some of them were about actual events. I treasured each and every story and, in my grandfather's honor, I try to pass them on," says Moore.

*Source: Tasks of Problem Solving, stories by LinguiSystems, 1992.

Moore invites the public to her store on Saturdays to hear stories of Johnny Appleseed, Paul Bunyan, and Davy Crockett. Go to her shop on Tuesdays and she'll spin tales of the Old West. According to customers, having Elsie pull the wool over your eyes is always a special treat.

Snowstorm Curbs Vacation Plans

HOUSTON, Texas—This time of year, many snowbirds flock to Texas to escape the cold winter weather in the north. Warm weather activities like boating, fishing, swimming, and tennis are normally a good bet for a winter holiday in Texas. Not this weekend!

Yesterday's sudden blizzard caught Texas and the weather forecasters by surprise. Severe winter weather had been predicted, but for states far to the north of Texas.

Both tourists and residents were forced to change plans for the holiday weekend because of the snow. Shoppers crowded stores to buy warm clothing, snow shovels, flashlights, and other storm-survival equipment.

Without snow-removal equipment, cities did what they could to keep traffic moving. Minor traffic accidents were reported across the state, and some motorists had to be rescued from drifts along the interstate highways.

Minor injuries resulting from traffic accidents caused a temporary strain on local hospitals, which had reduced staffs due to poor driving conditions. Officials say most hospitals are now back to normal operations.

Snowfall ranged from four to 12 inches, with the heaviest accumulations north of Houston. Forecasters say with normal temperatures expected later this week, the snow should melt rapidly.

A Texas native took the blizzard in stride saying, "That's just how we do things in Texas. If you're going to do something, do it big!"

Camp Connects Countries, Youth

SAN DIEGO, Calif.—Youth from around the world joined hands this week at the Countries United International Camp in San Diego. Young people ages 6 through 19 flew from all corners of the world to exchange ideas about international peace and cooperation. Their objective? To come up with ways to encourage peace in their home countries.

"I never thought I could make a difference in the world," said 11-year-old Kate Blaag of Denmark. "But now I know all our ideas will be shared with leaders around the world. Adults need to know how kids in the world feel about peaceful coexistence. We have fresh ideas and not a lot of prejudices."

Camp organizers said the week-long camp got youngsters involved in brainstorming, trust-building, and cultural recognition activities in addition to playing sports from around the world.

"I really learned a lot about working on a team," reported Shikeb Zaidi, 15, of Pakistan. "In my culture, men are taught to be leaders, to work alone, and to show strength. It was hard for me, at first, to remember to talk to my teammates to solve problems. But now I understand that many brains are better than one."

The 63 campers of Countries United International Camp seemed to agree on one thing as their last day approached...peace begins at home.

4

Advanced Cooperative Group Treatment for Individuals with Mild Aphasia

Penny Hatch

The purpose of this chapter is to describe the rationale, development, and implementation of advanced cooperative group treatment. This therapy approach is designed for mild aphasic clients who have experience in cooperative group treatment and require more advanced language practice. The goals are to improve the client's residual word-finding difficulties and to promote more complete discourse. In the case study presented throughout this chapter, the clinician used a narrative recall task with an emphasis on story grammar to achieve these goals. This format was selected because the narrative is a basic form of discourse that is familiar to all speakers. It has a clear organization of information and is presented in a chronological sequence. Additionally, narrative recall occurs frequently in daily communication, as speakers relate current and past life experiences to others.[1]

In cooperative group treatment, clients learn to select and recall key information from short stories. With advanced cooperative group treatment, clients learn to succinctly summarize and retell a longer, 300- to 500-word, story. Emphasis is placed on sequentially recalling story-grammar elements in a cohesive manner. According to Merritt and Liles,[2] a story grammar is the predictable pattern of organization used to express temporally and causally related information. Stein and

Table 4-1. Story Grammar Elements

Setting information: main character(s), time, location, and context

Initiating event: obstacle, moral dilemma, or problem

Internal response: plan devised by the main character(s) in response to the situation

Attempt: action(s) taken in an attempt to solve the problem

Direct consequence: the result of the attempt

Reaction: the character's response to what has occurred

Source: Modified from DD Merritt, BZ Liles. Story grammar ability in children with and without language disorder: Story generation, story retelling, and story comprehension. J Speech Hearing Res 1987;30:539.

Glenn[3] outlined a set of story grammar rules that include setting information, an initiating event, an internal response, an attempt, a direct consequence, and a reaction. A less detailed story grammar by Ulatowska and Chapman[1] described setting information, a complicating action, and a resolution. All of these elements must be included for a story recall to be complete. Definitions of story grammar elements are listed in Table 4-1.

While story recall is the specific task used in this therapy approach, the ultimate goal for the mild aphasic client is to improve discourse skills that are generalized beyond this format. The group setting allows clients to work as a team to complete the task. By working with a partner, clients gain additional skills, such as providing support and cueing for each other, developing problem-solving strategies, and evaluating group and individual performances.

Determining Which Clients to Group

Consideration of the following prerequisites is necessary when grouping clients for advanced cooperative group treatment:

- *Classification.* Aphasic clients should classify as anomic on the Western Aphasia Battery (WAB),[4] score within the high 80s to normal range, and exhibit residual word-finding difficulties. As indicated by the range of WAB scores, the client's general severity level must be mild. In some cases, individuals score within the normal range on a test like the WAB.

• *Prior group skills*. Individuals who participate at the advanced level of therapy need prior experience with cooperative group treatment to have experience cueing a partner.

• *Specific language skills*. Due to the nature of the task, participants must demonstrate adequate reading comprehension skills at the paragraph level. Auditory comprehension should range from normal to mildly impaired.

• *Motivation*. Willingness to work in a group is also prerequisite. The client's previous participation in cooperative group treatment and a desire to continue treatment demonstrate an interest in group therapy.

• *Common interests*. Common interests is an important prerequisite for story selection. Stories used in therapy should be interesting to both clients.

Baseline Assessment and Treatment Outcome Evaluation

A variety of measures can be used to establish baseline performance and to measure the effects of therapy over time. The following battery provides both impairment level and functional communication measures:

• WAB. The administration time is 60 minutes.

• Reading Comprehension Battery for Aphasia (RCBA).[5] The administration time is 60 minutes.

• American Speech-Language-Hearing Association Functional Assessment of Communication Skills for Adults (ASHA FACS).[6] No within-session time is used for this assessment. Scoring takes approximately 30 minutes of clinician time.

• Clinician-generated probes. The administration time is 15 minutes.

• Story-generation probe. The administration time is 5 minutes.

• Social-validation questionnaire. The administration time is 15 minutes (see Figure 4-3).

The case study described in this chapter consists of two mild aphasic individuals who will be referred to as LF and JG. Clinician-constructed probes were used to measure treatment effectiveness and generalization. These probes included two types of stories. The first story, *Mama's Memoirs* by Bailey White,[7] was a concrete narrative that contained explicit information. The second story, *The Scotty Who Knew Too Much*, a modern fable by James Thurber,[8] included more implicit information. During each probe, the client followed the written story as the clinician read aloud. Then, the client had 2 minutes to retell the story as completely as possible. The clinician informed the client that no help could be provided during the probes.

The story generalization probe focused on story generation. In therapy, clients worked on improving story-recall skills. With this generalization probe, LF and JG were required to apply story-recall skills to generate an original story from a picture. They looked at a picture and had 2 minutes to create a story about it. The clinician selected Norman Rockwell's *Easter Morning* for this task, which depicts a man reading the newspaper in his pajamas as his family appears to be leaving the house for church services.

Baseline performance was determined by administering each probe three times before starting treatment. Additionally, the clinician administered probes following every fourth session during treatment and at the conclusion of therapy.

Probe scores consisted of two separate percentages. The first score reflected the percentage of story-grammar elements reported by the client. The second score represented the percentage of reported story-grammar elements that was accurate and complete. For example, LF described an attempt made by one of the story characters but referred to the character as "her" without establishing a prior referent. In this case, LF received credit for reporting the particular story-grammar element (i.e., the first percentage), but the ambiguous pronoun did not qualify as accurate and complete (i.e., the second percentage). This method of scoring allowed the clinician to compare the use of story grammar to the client's complete and accurate recall skills.

Advance preparation of a tally sheet simplified probe scoring (see Figures 4-1 and 4-2 for sample tally sheets). Story-grammar elements were listed in the vertical column, and administration dates were listed horizontally. The clinician marked off previously determined story-grammar elements as the client reported them. When the client reported an element inaccurately or incompletely, the clinician indicated this by placing an *i*, rather than a +, next to the element. The number of reported elements was divided by the total number of predetermined story-grammar elements and multiplied by 100 to get a percentage. Next, this calculation procedure was repeated by comparing the number of accurately reported elements to the total number of elements reported by the client.

The Scotty Who Knew Too Much			
Date	4/2	4/4	4/6
Characters			
Scotty	+	+	+
Farm Dog	+	+	+
Skunk	+	+	+
Porcupine	–	–	i
Setting			
Farm	+	+	+
Woods	+	+	+
Initiating event			
Scotty bragged that he could beat anyone	+	+	+
Internal response			
Farm Dog tested Scotty by challenging him to fight a skunk and a porcupine	i	i	–
Attempt			
Scotty fought skunk	+	–	+
Scotty fought porcupine	–	–	–
Scotty fought Farm Dog	–	–	–
Direct consequence			
Scotty lost all three fights	i	–	i
Reaction			
Scotty went to a nursing home	–	–	–
Total story grammar elements reported (complete plus incomplete)	9 of 13	7 of 13	9 of 13
Percentage of 13 possible	69%	54%	69%
Total accurately reported story grammar elements	7 of 9	7 of 7	7 of 9
Percentage of reported elements that were accurate (complete elements divided by total elements reported)	78%	100%	78%

Figure 4-1. Sample probe score sheet for story recall. (– = omitted information; + = accurately reported information; i = incomplete.)

Easter Morning			
Date	4/2	4/4	4/9
Main characters			
Father	+	+	+
Mother	+	+	+
Children	+	+	+
Setting			
Home or living room	+	–	–
Time			
Easter or Sunday morning	+	+	+
Initiating event			
Time for church	+	+	+
Internal response			
Father does not want to go to church	+	–	+
Attempt			
Father hides in chair behind newspaper	–	–	–
Direct consequence			
Family leaves father behind	–	–	–
Reaction			
Family is angry at father, or father feels guilty	–	–	–
Total story-grammar elements reported (complete plus incomplete)	7 of 10	5 of 10	6 of 10
Percentage of 10 possible	70%	50%	60%
Total accurately reported story-grammar elements	7 of 7	5 of 5	6 of 6
Percentage of reported elements that were accurate (complete elements divided by total elements reported)	100%	100%	100%

Figure 4-2. Sample probe score sheet for story generation. (– = omitted information; + = accurately reported information; i = incomplete.)

1. Do you feel that you have made improvements by participating in this treatment?

2. If you feel that you made improvements, do you feel that it was worth the time and effort that you put into it?

3. Did you enjoy this therapy?

4. Would you recommend it to someone else who has similar language difficulties?

5. What was the worst part of this experience?

6. What was the best part of this experience?

7. Do you think working with a partner was helpful? If so, how do you think it helped?

8. Were there any disadvantages to working with a therapy partner?

9. Has this therapy had any impact on your communication or life outside the clinic?

10. Do you have any suggestions to improve this therapy approach?

Figure 4-3. Social validation questionnaire to be administered at the completion of therapy.

After completing all treatment sessions, the clinician administered and reviewed a social-validation questionnaire with each client and a family member or friend. Figure 4-3 is a sample questionnaire.

The Clinician's Task: Selecting the Goals or Objectives for the Group

As previously mentioned, the overall goal in advanced cooperative group treatment is improved discourse skills in mild aphasic clients. Several treatment objectives are included to achieve this goal.

Quantifiable Goals

1. *Improved story recall.* This goal is approached by determining and recalling pertinent information or story grammar elements. In narrative-recall tasks, clients must comprehend a story, mentally reorganize

and reduce the information, and restructure the information for discourse production.[9] Aphasic clients may have difficulty determining what information needs to be explained and what information can be implied. This results in the production of excessive detail.[10] Identifying and reporting story-grammar elements gives the client an approach to story recall that is complete and concise. To measure recall skills, the clinician determines the percentage of story-grammar elements reported by the client. These story-grammar elements are selected for each narrative by the clients with guidance from the clinician when necessary. The group cooperatively selects a limited number of events to summarize the story. Individual scores reflect the percentage of those events reported by each client during a 2-minute, noncued story recall. Both complete and incomplete reported elements are included in this score. For example, if the client reports an event but it contains an ambiguous reference or is out of sequence, the client receives credit for reporting the element. The clinician should, however, note that the element was incomplete. This information is used to determine the accuracy of reported elements score.

2. *Accurate story sequencing.* To achieve this, the clients select three or four elements from the beginning, middle, and end of the story and record them on a diagram that provides visual support (Figure 4-4).[11] After completing this task, the clients close their eyes and visualize the diagram as the clinician reads the story. During the story recall, the clinician removes the diagram; however, clients are encouraged to reconstruct a mental image of the diagram if it is helpful. Sequencing skills are measured during the 2-minute, noncued story recall. When clients report a story element out of sequence, it is an incomplete response. While the incomplete response is included in the percentage of reported elements, a separate percentage is calculated for the accuracy of reported elements. To determine this percentage, the clinician divides the number of accurate and complete reported elements by the total number of elements reported by the client (complete and incomplete) and multiplies by 100.

3. *Decreased use of ambiguous references.* Reference errors include the use of a referent without an antecedent or the use of an ambiguous referent.[1] When this occurs, it can be extremely difficult for the naïve listener to follow the events of a story. Treatment to improve complete and accurate recall includes increasing client awareness of errors and discussing the impact of those errors on story comprehension. The accuracy of reported elements score reflects the

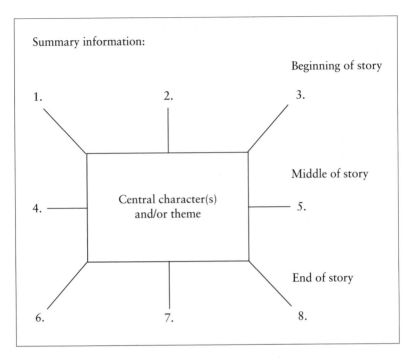

Figure 4-4. Story diagram.

client's referencing skills. Reported elements containing ambiguous references are scored as incomplete. As mentioned previously, incomplete elements are included in the percentage of elements reported; however, they lower the client's accuracy score.

4. *Improved word-finding skills.* The production of ambiguous referents and excessive detail can be a by-product of a word-retrieval deficit. Pronouns without prior referents can result from an inability to retrieve a specific name, or clients may provide unnecessary details to fill time when a particular story event is inaccessible. A variety of cueing strategies and visualization are used to improve word finding. Additionally, clients spend a few minutes doing deep-breathing exercises before unassisted story recalls. The goal of the deep breathing is to put the client in a calm and relaxed state. Informal observation during therapy sessions revealed that deep breathing and relaxation helped clients focus on the task and reportedly reduced anxiety when word-finding diffi-

culties occurred. Word-retrieval difficulties can affect both the percentage of reported elements and the accuracy of reported elements. For example, when clients have trouble retrieving a specific word or phrase, they use additional time trying to access this information. If the client spends too much time on this, the 2-minute time constraint prohibits recall of other known story-grammar elements. In addition, the client may report only the information about the element that is accessible, resulting in incomplete responses and a lower accuracy score.

Qualitative Goals

Additional therapy objectives relate to working in a group. Throughout treatment, progress is documented through clinician observation and client feedback.

1. *Increased understanding and use of cueing strategies.* Advanced cooperative group treatment participants develop and improve cueing strategies during their initial participation in cooperative group treatment. This therapy approach emphasizes effective cueing with progress monitored through scoring. Advanced cooperative treatment also requires clients to use cueing, but the primary goal of therapy is the production of a complete and sequential recall of the gist of a story. Evaluation of cueing performance and effective strategies is informal, consisting of clinician observation and client feedback.

2. *Development of problem-solving skills.* Clients develop problem-solving skills by discussing areas of difficulty and working cooperatively to develop solutions. The client typically recommends strategies that he or she has found helpful and makes suggestions based on observations of his or her partner's recall.

3. *Improved ability to evaluate individual and group performance.* This skill is developed through a discussion that concludes every session. Clients evaluate their own performance as well as the performance of the group. Discussions focus on specific areas of difficulty and highlight successful strategies and improvements. Areas for improvement may include increasing objective observation skills, decreasing self-criticism, and increasing the client's willingness to offer constructive criticism.

4. *Refinement of negotiating skills.* As clients become comfortable with their partners and more confident in their skills, they learn to work as a team. Through the cooperative selection of story-grammar elements, clients develop the ability to defend their choices, exercise their rights as group members, and negotiate solutions when a difference of opinion occurs.

5. *Development of trust.* Once clients gain a sense of trust in the group, they frequently share common experiences and coping strategies. Aphasic clients often provide insight to their therapy partners that the nonaphasic clinician cannot. In this sense, the clients are the experts and they become the providers, rather than the receivers, of information.

Five-Step Treatment Process

Before beginning therapy, the clinician assesses each client individually, introduces the group members, and explains the treatment goals. After completing this, the group begins work on the specific therapy task. Clients summarize and recall treatment stories, and at the end of each session their performances are scored. Additionally, the clinician administers generalization probes after every fourth session.

The primary treatment materials used in advanced cooperative group treatment are narrative stories that are 300–500 words in length. Story topics and sources should reflect the clients' interests. For example, LF and JG were San Francisco 49ers football fans. The clinician found a book composed of short stories that recounted the history of the team.[12] LF and JG enjoyed these stories, which resulted in improved performance scores. Stories about current events or celebrities are also interesting to most clients and can be found in sources such as *People* magazine.

The clinician's role in helping attain the therapy goals changes throughout treatment. Initially, the clinician directs the sessions, teaching clients how to cue each other, and helps select information for the story diagram. As treatment progresses, the clinician provides direction and support only when needed. For example, rather than telling group members specifically when and how to cue their partner, the clinician might provide a prompt by suggesting that a cue would be helpful. The clinician also becomes less involved in the selection of story recall elements. Rather than suggesting specific elements, the clinician might assist only in negotiations or disagreements about what to include. The clinician's final role is to observe the entire cueing and recall process and participate only during the review of the session.

Assessment (Sessions 1 and 2)

As mentioned in "Baseline Assessment and Treatment Outcome Evaluation," the assessment battery includes the WAB, RCBA, and ASHA FACS. To establish baseline performance, the client also completes three treatment and generalization probes before starting therapy. Individual assessment typically requires about 2.0–2.5 hours per client.

Getting to Know the Clients (Session 3)

In the first group treatment session, the clinician introduces the clients and briefly reviews the story-recall format. Next, the clients discuss topics of interest and possible story sources. Occasionally, clients say that they do not have a particular area of interest and that any subject is fine. In this case, the clinician should offer several topics and ask the clients to choose one.

Discussing the Goals of Treatment (Sessions 3 and 4)

The clinician reviews the story-recall task and relates this to the overall goal of improved conversational skills. Occurrences of story recall in everyday conversation should be emphasized. Examples of conversational recall could include summarizing daily events, describing a vacation, or retelling an amusing family story. The clinician should also discuss specific objectives such as improved word finding and story sequencing. Next, the clinician explains the concept of story grammar and how to use this as a framework for developing a story diagram and effectively retelling a story. The clinician should list and define the various story grammar elements and explain how the inclusion of each element creates a complete story. (One example of story grammar elements is listed in Table 4-1 and is based on the work of Merritt and Liles.[2]) A review of group goals includes discovering and using facilitating cues, negotiating the selection of story elements, and evaluating group and individual performances. The clinician also informs the clients that they will gradually receive less assistance and eventually take over the role of the clinician.

Stories (Sessions 4–17)

Each story proceeds through the following sequence:

1. *Reading the story.* The first 300- to 500-word story is introduced. Both clients read silently as the clinician reads the story aloud.

2. *Creating the story diagram.* The group members divide the story into three sections—beginning, middle, and end.[11] They select a central story character, theme, or event to be placed in the middle of the diagram. Next, the group determines two or three events that occurred in each part of the story and writes them on the story diagram. The beginning section of the story often includes the names of important characters, a setting, and an initiating event. The middle section usually includes an attempt, and the end section typically contains the result of the attempt and the character's response. Figure 4-5 is a sample story diagram that was created to summarize a story from *People* magazine. The group reviews the story one or two paragraphs at a time while creating the diagram. Initially, the clinician helps the clients with this task. As therapy progresses, the clients should become more independent in selecting these elements. Clients should be encouraged to express opinions about the information selected for the diagram, defend personal selections, and negotiate solutions to disagreements. After completing the diagram, each client takes a few minutes to study it.

3. *Rereading the story.* The story diagram is placed in the center of the table. As the clinician rereads the story, the clients close their eyes and try to visually follow the path of the story diagram.

4. *Cooperative story recall.* The clients take turns recalling sections of the story. For example, the first client describes the beginning, the second client recalls the middle, and the first client describes the story's ending. If a client experiences difficulty, his or her partner is free to provide any type of cueing. After completing the story, the group evaluates each client's performance and does any necessary problem solving to improve the recall of missed elements. Next, the clients repeat the cooperative recall with the other client starting the process. Group evaluation and problem solving follow the second recall. Examples of problem solving include suggestions to recall the story at a slower pace, visualizing the diagram while mentally "walking along the path of the story," and using a specific type of self-cueing.

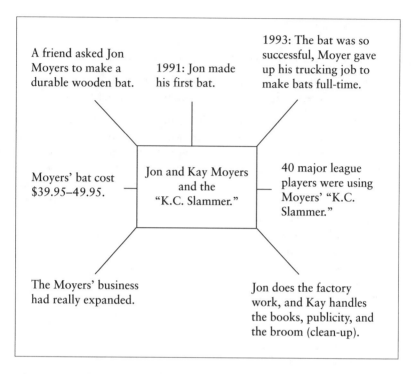

A friend asked Jon Moyers to make a durable wooden bat.

1991: Jon made his first bat.

1993: The bat was so successful, Moyer gave up his trucking job to make bats full-time.

Moyers' bat cost $39.95–49.95.

Jon and Kay Moyers and the "K.C. Slammer."

40 major league players were using Moyers' "K.C. Slammer."

The Moyers' business had really expanded.

Jon does the factory work, and Kay handles the books, publicity, and the broom (clean-up).

Figure 4-5. Sample story diagram. This diagram summarizes a story from *People* magazine about a husband and wife from Kansas City. The couple had a friend who asked them to make a durable baseball bat for his amateur team. The bat caught the attention of several professional baseball players and became popular, resulting in the development of a successful company.

5. *Breathing (optional).* During one problem-solving discussion, the clinician suggested this relaxation exercise to improve word recall. After trying it, the clients asked to include it as a step in therapy. Before the final story recall, the clients should close their eyes and spend a few minutes deep breathing. The clinician encourages the clients to slowly breathe in, pause at the top of the breath, and very slowly release the air. Once the clients are relaxed, the clinician reads the story one final time.

6. *Individual story recall.* A group typically completes one story per session. After practice has been completed, each client has 2 minutes to independently retell the story. During this time, no cueing is pro-

vided. Clients alternate between the roles of recaller and listener for a single story. When acting as the listener, the client observes his or her partner's performance and develops constructive criticism. Recall scores represent the percentage of elements recalled from the group-generated story diagram. If a portion of a reported element is ambiguous or incomplete, this should be documented. The percentage of elements recalled includes both complete and incomplete elements. To obtain the accuracy of recalled elements score, the clinician divides the number of completely reported elements by the total number of reported elements and multiplies that number by 100. Although the clients are not trying to identify specific story-grammar elements, they are typically included in the story diagram to facilitate a complete and concise story recall.

7. *Post-story recall evaluation.* After completing the individual story recall, each client evaluates his or her, as well as his or her partner's, performance. The group discusses specific problems and exchanges ideas for potential solutions. The evaluation also includes a critique of the elements selected for the story diagram. Were these selections truly representative of the story? Did they facilitate a comprehensive but concise story recall? The group's observations of what worked and what did not are incorporated into the next story sequence.

8. *Generalization probes.* After every fourth session, the clinician administers probes to assess the effects of treatment and generalization.

9. *Homework.* One homework suggestion is to send home a copy of the treatment story for the next session. This gives the clients an opportunity to familiarize themselves with the story. Another suggestion is to have clients keep a journal of their communication experiences. A journal review is a good way to start each session. Clients can record and discuss communication successes, failures, and fears, while the group atmosphere provides encouragement and support.

After completing all treatment sessions, the clinician administers a final treatment and generalization probe and reviews a social validation questionnaire (see Figure 4-3).

Discharge (Session 18)

The final session includes a review of outcome data and a discussion of improvements and future goals. The clinician also provides a home program. Activities should be similar to those practiced in therapy and appropriate for clients to complete independently. For example, clients could audiotape themselves while retelling a treatment story. Then, they could listen to the taped recall, using the previously completed story diagram to evaluate their performance. Appendix 4A describes sample home program activities.

On the final day of therapy, the clinician also administers and reviews a social validation questionnaire with the client and a family member or friend (see Figure 4-3). Administering the questionnaire separately to each client provides the necessary privacy to express any dissatisfaction or discomfort with the group experience. Interviewing a family member or friend, in addition to the client, provides the clinician with more information about the client's communication changes outside the clinic.

Example of a Typical Session

This session occurred after approximately fifteen treatment sessions. The story came from *People* magazine. It described a married couple from Kansas City who created a durable baseball bat as a favor for a friend. Several professional baseball players discovered and began using the bat, resulting in the development of a successful company (see Figure 4-5). After reading the story, LF and JG selected three events to summarize the beginning of the story and two summary events for both the middle and the end of the story. Without specifically identifying story grammar elements (i.e., a setting, a complicating action, and a resolution), the clients naturally included them in their story diagram. They individually studied the diagram and then tried to visually recreate it, as the clinician reread the story. During the cooperative recall, LF had difficulty remembering one of the beginning elements. Her partner, JG, effectively cued her by asking a leading question (i.e., "Why did Jon Moyer make his first baseball bat?"). The cooperative recalls were followed by deep breathing and individual story recalls with no cueing provided. Both clients accurately reported six of the seven selected story elements. Although the group members were generally satisfied with their performance, the evaluation revealed some constructive criticism for JG. He began to rush through the end of the story and left out one important detail. During the next session, he incorporated this information by making an effort to remain calm. This resulted in a perfect recall score.

Case Example

LF, a 64-year-old woman, had a left posterior cerebral artery aneurysm and subarachnoid hemorrhage approximately 1 year before participating in advanced cooperative group treatment. She consistently received speech-language therapy following her cerebrovascular accident and had previously completed two quarters of cooperative group treatment. LF's assessment revealed an Aphasia Quotient of 90.9 (normal cut-off 93.8) on the WAB and RCBA scores ranging from 60% to 100%. She demonstrated moderate reading comprehension at the paragraph level. Her performance on the ASHA FACS indicated effective, independent communication of basic needs and wants with minimal assistance required for social communication. LF's mean baseline score for reported story grammar elements in the narrative probe was 45% with 79% accuracy. The mean baseline score for the fable was 43% for elements reported with 71% accuracy. Her mean baseline score for the story generation probe was 54% for reported story grammar elements with 100% accuracy.

General behavioral observations revealed a motivated and diligent client. During the previous two quarters of cooperative group treatment, LF had developed greater self-confidence and began to be less self-critical. At the beginning of advanced cooperative group treatment, she frequently expressed concern regarding her performance (e.g., "I hope I'm doing this right") but appeared more confident and relaxed in testing situations.

Although the advanced cooperative group therapy sessions were challenging for LF, she seemed motivated rather than discouraged by the challenge. Poor performance during a cooperative recall consistently resulted in improvements during the individual, noncued recall. Additionally, LF did not hesitate to exercise her rights as a group member. She asked for help or clarification when she needed it. She contributed to the story diagrams with minimal or no prompting and appropriately defended her selection of story elements.

At the completion of therapy, LF's mean probe scores for reported elements reflected her improvement. Her mean pre- and post-treatment probe scores increased from 45% to 56% on the narrative and 43% to 67% on the fable. The mean score for reported elements in the story generation from the Norman Rockwell picture increased from 54% at baseline to 63% after treatment. The mean score for the accuracy of reported elements remained stable or decreased slightly.

LF completed a social-validation questionnaire during her final therapy session. She reported that she had enjoyed participating in advanced cooperative group treatment and that she would "highly recommend it" to other aphasic individuals with similar language difficulties. Additionally, LF reported that her success in therapy had increased her self-confidence. As a result, she had recently returned to her church for the first time since her cerebrovascular accident. LF's husband reported that his wife was now having less word-finding difficulty and that she had increased her use of telephone communication. For example, she independently arranged to have the roof repaired and made hotel reservations over the phone.

Important Points About This Treatment

The following points should be considered when using advanced cooperative group treatment:

• When selecting stories, it is important that they are interesting to the clients. Encourage clients, their family members, and friends to participate in the story-selection process.

• The story diagram facilitates the development of negotiation skills. As therapy progresses, the clients improve their ability to justify their individual selections and to work out compromises when disagreements occur.

• The evaluation portion of the session is an important component of this group treatment. In this format, clients learn how to encourage each other and how to provide constructive criticism. They also develop their own problem-solving strategies and often give the clinician valuable insight into the client's language and problem-solving difficulties.

Common Questions and Solutions

Question: What if the task is too difficult for the client?
Answer: If the initial task seems too difficult for the client, provide support by using multiple modalities. For example, the story diagram was originally incorporated into the therapy task to help JG who was struggling with the story recall. The diagram helped him visualize the story and limited the amount of information that he could

select for the recall. In previous sessions, JG had tried to recall the story in too much detail, which affected his performance. The story diagram helped him summarize the story, using a limited amount of pertinent information. Task difficulty can also be varied through story selection. Begin therapy with concrete stories that contain explicit information (e.g., biographical articles). To make the task harder, progress to stories that contain implied information (e.g., fables, short mystery stories).

Question: What should the clinician do when one group member is more successful than the other?

Answer: One inevitable difficulty of working in a dyad is comparison between group members. Although the group can work together to develop strategies, the less-successful client may become discouraged. One successful solution to this problem includes focusing on a specific area for each client to improve while making slight accommodations for the client who has difficulty. For example, JG became anxious during his timed story recall. When timed, he had more word-finding difficulty than usual and consistently ran out of time before completing the story. The clinician worked with JG to include only the most important information in his recall and temporarily removed the time constraint. While JG continued his story until he was finished, the clinician quietly stopped scoring after the 2-minute time limit ended. Eventually, JG developed confidence in his ability to successfully perform the task and was not bothered by the time constraint. This temporary accommodation helped JG improve both his self-confidence and his performance.

Question: What if one or both clients are not interested in the therapy stories?

Answer: One way to avoid this problem is to select stories based on client interests. The clinician should discuss this with clients during the initial treatment session or send home a questionnaire before starting therapy. Sometimes clients say that they do not have a particular area of interest. In this case, the clinician can offer some suggestions (e.g., sports, current events, history, biographies, travel). Additionally, clients and their families should be encouraged to participate in the story-selection process. For homework, ask each client to bring in one short newspaper or magazine article to be used in therapy. In case they forget, the clinician should always bring three or four stories about different subjects. If the clients do not have any common areas of interest (e.g., one client likes sports and the other likes fashion), the clinician can alternate story topics. The clinician may even find a story that incorporates both subjects (e.g., a clothing line put out by a popular sports figure). The therapy situation is ideal when both clients have a common interest and the clinician is not well informed about the topic. In addition to making the sessions more interesting, this gives the clients a chance to share their expertise with the less-knowledgeable clinician.

Question: What if the group is not completing the task quickly enough?

Answer: Creating the story diagram is usually the most time-consuming part of the therapy task. One way to move through this more quickly is to send the therapy story home and have clients read it before the session. Another way to speed up the diagramming process is to have a time limit. If clients are having difficulty agreeing on what information to include, and this is using up too much time, suggest that the clients alternate when providing information. For example, one client can select the central story theme and the other can list the beginning story elements. While it is important for clients to learn negotiation skills, it is also important to have enough therapy time to practice re-telling the story and to evaluate the group's performance.

Recommended Sources for Materials

Any 300- to 500-word story that interests the clients can be used in advanced cooperative group treatment. Newspaper or magazine articles are excellent sources. Suggested magazines include *People*, *Reader's Digest*, and *Sports Illustrated*. One advantage to *Reader's Digest* is that it is easy to obtain large-print copies. If print size is a consideration for group members, many photocopiers can enlarge print. The clinician used several collections of short stories. These included *Mama Makes Up Her Mind* by Bailey White,[7] *The Thurber Carnival* by James Thurber,[8] and *San Francisco 49ers: The First Fifty Years* by Glenn Dickey.[12] Finally, it is important to consider that concrete and explicit stories are easier for clients to recall than stories with implied information (e.g., fables). The difficulty level of the therapy task can be modified by altering the story choices and by increasing the amount of multimodality support and clinician input.

References

1. Ulatowska HK, Chapman SB. Discourse Studies. In R Lubinski (ed), Dementia and Communication. Philadelphia: BC Decker, 1991;115.
2. Merritt DD, Liles BZ. Story grammar ability in children with and without language disorder: Story generation, story retelling, and story comprehension. J Speech Hearing Res 1987;30:539.
3. Stein NL, Glenn CG. An Analysis of Story Comprehension in Elementary School Children. In RO Freedle (ed), New Directions in Discourse Processing. Norwood, NJ: Ablex, 1979;53.
4. Kertesz A. Western Aphasia Battery. New York: Grune & Stratton, 1982.
5. LaPointe L, Horner J. Reading Comprehension Battery for Aphasia. Tigard, OR: CC Publications, 1979.
6. Frattali C, Thompkins C, Holland A, et al. Functional Assessment of Communication Skills for Adults. Rockville, MD: ASHA, 1995.
7. White B. Mama Makes Up Her Mind and Other Dangers of Southern Living. New York: Vintage Books, 1993.
8. Thurber J. The Thurber Carnival. New York: Harper & Row, 1954.
9. Ulatowska HK, Chapman SB. Discourse Macrostructure in Aphasia. In R Bloom, L Obler, S DeSanti, J Erlich (eds), Discourse Analysis and Applications. Hillsdale, NJ: Lawrence Erlbaum Associates, 1994;29.
10. Chapman SB, Ulatowska HK. Methodology for discourse management in the treatment of aphasia. Clin Communication Disord 1992;2:64.
11. Ford J. Personal communication, 1996. The Aphasia Center, Texas Women's University Dallas Center, Parkland Campus.
12. Dickey G. San Francisco 49ers: The First Fifty Years. Atlanta: Turner Publishing, 1995.

Appendix 4A:
Home Program

General Directions

The following activities are exercises from previous therapy sessions. These activities are provided to help maintain and increase the story-summary skills that were acquired during treatment. Find a quiet room where you can work without any interruptions. Work on one of the activities listed below at least three times a week. You should spend 20–30 minutes on each activity.

Specific Instructions

Story-Recall Practice

You will need a tape recorder and an audiotape for this activity. Enclosed are five stories and story diagrams that we worked on in therapy. Select and read one of the stories. For example, read the story that describes how George Seifert was hired as head coach of the San Francisco 49ers. When you are finished, review the completed story summary diagram. It shows a central theme or character (e.g., George

Seifert becomes head coach of the 49ers) and two or three events that occurred in the beginning, middle, and end of the story. After reviewing the diagram, close your eyes for a few moments as you take several deep breaths. Visualize the summary diagram and mentally walk yourself along the story's path, from beginning to end. Next, tape yourself as you retell the story. Rewind the tape and listen to yourself. As you listen, use the diagram to check off each of the characters and events that you mentioned. Check for any information that was omitted from your recall. When you have successfully recalled all or most of the events and characters in the story diagram, you should progress to "Telling a Story to a Listener."

Telling a Story to a Listener

This activity requires a partner and a tape recorder. Use the stories and summary diagrams that you used in "Story-Recall Practice." I have also provided you with an inventory "List of Potential Listener Questions" that your listening partner might ask. This will help you track patterns of omitted information. As in "Story-Recall Practice," begin by reading the story and reviewing the summary diagram. Take a few moments to breathe deeply and visualize the diagram before you recall the story. Next, audio-tape yourself as you tell the story to a listener. After you have finished, ask your listener if he or she has any questions. Use the inventory sheet that I have provided to keep track of the types of questions asked (e.g., Who did that happen to? or Why did that person go there?). Before you recall your next story, pay particular attention to the areas that were omitted in your previous recall. Remember, however, that sometimes listeners forget information that has been mentioned. If your listener asked a question about information that you mentioned, do not mark it on the question sheet. Finally, listen to the audiotape of the recall and evaluate your own performance.

Optional Activity

I have also enclosed three new stories and blank story diagrams. These stories are similar to those that we worked on in therapy (e.g., 49ers history, articles about current events, short biographical stories about celebrities). You can use them for "Story-Recall Practice" and "Telling a Story to a Listener" if you would like extra practice, but you will need to fill in the story diagram on your own.

Reading Journal

This activity is designed to help you apply the story-summary skills that we worked on to your own reading. Select a book that interests you. Start your journal by summarizing a few pages at a time. Try to limit your entries to four or five written statements. Gradually increase the amount of material that you summarize, eventually working up to a chapter. I have enclosed a "List of Questions for the Reading Journal" to help you summarize the information. If you find the questions helpful, refer to them when writing your summary. After you have finished the book, read your journal and see how well it summarizes the story.

Personal Journal

Finally, continue to keep your personal journal. Try to record two or three activities each day. This gives you practice writing and is a good way to document communication challenges and successes.

List of Potential Listener Questions

1. Who was this story about?
2. Who did a particular action?
3. Why did a character do a particular action?
4. Where did this story take place?
5. When did an event happen?
6. What is the main problem in this story?
7. What did the character(s) do to handle a particular problem?
8. Was the character successful in the attempt to solve the problem?
9. How did the story end?
10. How did the character(s) feel about the outcome?

List of Questions for the Reading Journal

1. Who were the characters in this passage?
2. Was the time or place mentioned or important in this passage?
3. Was there a particular problem that the character(s) encountered?
4. What actions did the character(s) take to handle the problem?
5. Do you know the outcome of those actions?
6. How did the character(s) react to the events of the story?

5

Modified Cooperative Group Treatment for Individuals with Moderate Aphasia

Elizabeth L. Hoover

The purpose of this chapter is to describe a variation of cooperative group treatment designed to increase functional communication skills for moderately impaired aphasic individuals. A case study involving two moderately aphasic individuals (CB and SV) is provided throughout the chapter to illustrate this approach. Aphasia disrupts the integrity of the whole person and causes long-term effects on lifestyle and environment.[1] Augmentative and alternative communication devices for use with aphasia is an attempt to increase communicative effectiveness in light of long-term deficits.[1] This treatment incorporates the development and use of a communication notebook as augmentative communication to that end. Treatment was provided twice weekly for 2 weeks (including four individual sessions for baseline testing).

Determining Which Clients to Group

Grouping of clients was determined by the following:

- *Classification.* Group members should have similar etiologies. Both group members (CB and SV) were classified with Broca's aphasia and obtained an Aphasia Quotient of 65–70 on the Western Aphasia Battery.[2]

• *Specific language skills.* Group members should have comparable or complementary strengths and weaknesses. In the case study, both group members were able to read minimally at the five- or six-word sentence level, demonstrated relatively strong auditory comprehension skills (i.e., were able to process two to three units of information), had limited verbal expression (i.e., less than four words per utterance), and had limited writing abilities (i.e., one to three words per sentence).

• *Motivation.* Ideally, group members should show interest and enthusiasm in the cooperative group process. During the treatment discussed herein, motivation appeared directly linked to the amount of time spent practicing and the few absences seen throughout the treatment. As the group progressed, it tended to take on a personality of its own; the group became more enthusiastic and looked forward to attending and participating in treatment.

• *Common interests.* As with any social group, members with some common interests and compatible personalities make the dynamic of the group more natural. CB and SV shared several interests, which made finding appropriate themes and topics for the treatment activities much easier.

• Criteria not used for grouping clients in this treatment included gender, education, and time postonset.

Assessment and Treatment Outcome Measures

Baseline Testing

Several tests and clinician-generated treatment probes were used to establish baseline performance and to provide a means to evaluate treatment outcome. Each client was tested individually.

• Western Aphasia Battery.[1] The administration time was 50–60 minutes.

• Reading Comprehension Battery for Aphasia.[3] The administration time was 1.5 hours.

- American Speech-Language-Hearing Association Functional Assessment of Communication Skills for Adults (ASHA FACS).[4] The administration required no in-session time; however, 20–30 minutes of clinician time was required.

- Motor speech evaluation.[5] The administration time was 20 minutes.

- Treatment probes. The administration time varied from 5 to 20 minutes for each story.

Treatment probes were designed and administered before treatment to obtain baseline data and to track generalization to untreated tasks throughout therapy. The probe consisted of three 75- to 80-word short stories each with five to six comprehension questions and was administered three times before treatment (see Appendix 5A). During the probe administration, the client was asked to follow the short story as it was read aloud by the clinician. The client was then asked to answer the comprehension questions either verbally, gesturally, in writing, or by underlining the appropriate answer in the body of the text. Next, the client was asked to retell the story using any communication modality as completely as possible. Performance was scored for accuracy using modified Porch Index of Communicative Ability (PICA)[6] scoring, communicative gist, and the rate of information communicated per minute (ipm). Modality (i.e., verbal, written, or gestural) was analyzed independent of accuracy. The modified PICA scoring system is based on the 16-point rating scale designed by Porch.[6] It was used to assign a severity score for each communication attempt based on its accuracy, promptness, efficiency, and complexity (Table 5-1).[6] Each score greater than ten (scores of 11 or higher have no inaccurate information) was divided by the total number of utterances and converted to a percentage to give a communicative gist score. Each story retell was timed and a ratio of the amount of information conveyed (by any modality) per minute was calculated to determine the rate of output. Figure 5-1 provides an example of a story, comprehension questions, and story retell complete with scoring.

Treatment Outcome Measures

Treatment outcome was evaluated through three methods: daily data collection, generalization probes, and social validation.

Table 5-1. The Porch Index of Communicative Ability Categories
for Scoring Responses

Score	Category	Dimensional Characteristics
16	Complex	Accurate, responsive, complex, prompt, efficient
15	Complete	Accurate, responsive, complex, prompt, efficient
14	Distorted	Accurate, responsive, complete or complex, distorted
13	Complete-delayed	Accurate, responsive, complete or complex, delayed
12	Incomplete	Accurate, responsive, incomplete, prompt
11	Incomplete-delayed	Accurate, responsive, incomplete, delayed
10	Corrected	Accurate, self-corrected
9	Repeated	Accurate (after instructions are repeated)
8	Cued	Accurate (after cue is given)
7	Related	Inaccurate, almost accurate
6	Error	Inaccurate attempt at the task item
5	Intelligible	Comprehensible but not an attempt at the task item
4	Unintelligible	Incomprehensible but differentiated
3	Minimal	Incomprehensible and undifferentiated
2	Attention	No response; patient attends to the tester
1	No response	No awareness of task

Source: Reprinted with permission from B Porch. The Porch Index of Communicative Ability. Austin, TX: PRO-ED, 1981.

Daily Data Collection

The clinician recorded all group-communicated information on line (as it was attempted) and assigned a modified PICA score to each utterance (see Table 5-1). A mean accuracy and range of scores was calculated from the PICA scores, as well as a communicative gist score and rate of communicative content per minute. In addition, each utterance was assigned a prefix, W (written), G (gestural), or V (verbal), to calculate the percentage of modalities used. An example of an on-line daily probe based on the story about CB's schedule is in Figure 5-2.

CB's Schedule

CB gets up at about 8:30 or 9:00 AM
He washes, dresses, and then eats breakfast.
Monday, Wednesday, and Thursday mornings, he goes to his PE class at Chabot College.
Lunch is at noon, when he watches *Days of Our Lives.*
Tuesday, Wednesday, and Thursday afternoons, CB comes to Cal State Hayward for therapy.
Dinner is usually around 6:00 PM
He goes to bed at 11:00 PM
(74 words)

Questions	Accuracy Score	Gist Score
When does CB get up?	15	+
Which days does he go to Chabot College?	12	+
What happens at noon?	12	+
Which days does CB come to Cal State Hayward?	12	+
What time is dinner?	15	+
What time does he go to bed?	12	+
Average accuracy score ($\overline{X}$) and percentage gist score	$\overline{X}$ = 13 (78/6) Range = 12–15 of accuracy scores	100% (6/6)

Figure 5-1. Sample story and questions with baseline scores.

Score	Modality	Communication
12	Verbal	Chuck
6	Verbal	Cal State Hayward
10	Written	Chabot
7	Gestural	Monday Wednesday Friday
12	Written	Physical therapy
12	Verbal and gestural	Lunch noon *Days of Lives*
7	Verbal	Chuck dinner 7 PM
10	Written	6:00 PM
12	Gestural	Bed 11:00 PM
6	Verbal	Goodnight
12	Verbal	Cal State Wednesday
7	Gestural	Monday Wednesday Friday
6	Gestural	Tuesday Wednesday Friday
6	Gestural	Monday Wednesday
11	Verbal	8:30 AM
11	Gestural	Wash
11	Gestural	Breakfast

158

37 units of information (U of I) ÷ 3 minutes = 12.3. 12.3 ÷ 3 = 4.1 U of I communicated per minute (average).

$\overline{X}$ = 9.3, range = 6–12, >10: 8÷17 (47%).

Figure 5-2. Example of an on-line daily probe. Three minutes were required for administration of this probe. The sum of PICA$_6$ severity scores (for each utterance is S158) is divided by the number of communicative utterances (17) to get the mean accuracy score ($\overline{X}$ = 9.3) + the overall range of severity scores (r = 6–12). Communicative gist is calculated by tallying the number of severity scores greater than 10 and dividing that number by the total number of utterances (>10: 8÷17 or 47%).

Generalization

To measure generalization of treatment, each group member's performance was probed every fourth session (i.e., bimonthly). Clients were seen individually and outside of the scheduled cooperative group treatment. Each probe session lasted from 30 minutes to 1 hour, as individual performance varied. The order of the probe stories was determined by the client; therefore, presentation order varied from session to session. Probe administration closely followed the daily cooperative group treatment. For example, after the story order was chosen, the story was read aloud by the clinician as the client followed along. Next, the client completed the comprehension questions, by either verbalizing, writing, or gesturing the answer. (Pointing to the answer in the body of the text was scored as a gestural response.) Then the client recalled the story using any communication modality. Pen, paper, and the client's communication notebook were provided to aid communication. Scoring procedures were identical to those described in the section on daily data collection.

Social Validation

Social validation measures were taken at the end of treatment to determine the client's opinions about the appropriateness and value of treatment. Questionnaires were used with a seven-point rating scale to enable the clients to fill out the forms independently.

The Clinician's Task: Selecting the Goals or Objectives for the Group

The overall objective for this cooperative group treatment was to increase functional discourse for both group members. This was accomplished through the following quantifiable and qualitative goals:

Quantifiable Goals

1. The client will increase the accuracy and amount of informational content via verbal, written, and gestural modalities produced during story-recall tasks (treatment and generalization probes) as measured by a modified PICA scoring system.

2. The client will increase his or her use of appropriate cueing when acting as the facilitator during a cooperative-therapy task, as measured by clinician observation and client feedback.

Qualitative Goals

1. The client will participate in the development and use of a communication notebook to facilitate self-cueing and word retrieval abilities, as evaluated by clinician observation and client feedback.

2. The client and caregiver will complete a social-validation questionnaire, using a seven-point rating scale, to determine their opinions on the appropriateness and value of this treatment (see Appendixes 5B and 5C).

Treatment

Treatment for the moderately impaired group differed from the original cooperative group treatment in one important way: the development and use of a communication notebook. To ensure that the communication notebook best met the needs of the group members, it was necessary to find out their individual interests and select functional communication topics and settings. This was accomplished by sending home an environmental questionnaire that was completed by the client and spouse and returned before treatment (see Appendix 5D).

Based on the clients' collective interests, the communication notebook was divided into nine sections: (1) notepaper and alphabet board, (2) biographical information, (3) maps, (4) "About My Stroke," (5) time, (6) numbers and money, (7) common phrases, (8) hobbies, and (9) foods. An 8 × 5.5–inch three-ring binder was chosen to house the notebook because of its convenient size and ability to add new pages. In addition, many datebooks or organizers on the market, such as Filofax or Dayrunner, use this size and format; therefore, the communication notebook can easily be transferred to an alternate binder if desired by the client.

One section was added to the communication book per week through the use of 75- to 85-word short stories. The majority of the stories were written using simple declarative sentences based on the reading comprehension levels of the group members. Two to three stories, using the information provided in the questionnaire (see Appendix 5D), were used to introduce each topic. For example, the "about my stroke" section was introduced in the third week through two stories: *What Is Aphasia* and *About Our Strokes* (see Appendix 5E). Visual aids, such as an anterior-posterior view of the left hemisphere of the brain for the *What Is Aphasia* story, were provided with the stories to aid comprehension. Initially, all stories were typed in enlarged font, with each sentence printed on a new line to aid reduced reading comprehension. As the treatment progressed, this was unnecessary, and the sentences were provided in a single paragraph.

Step One: Assessment (Sessions 1 to 4)

Each client was assessed individually, according to the assessment battery described in "Assessment and Treatment Outcome Measures." The entire assessment was completed over four 1-hour sessions.

Step Two: Getting to Know the Group Members (Session 5)

The first treatment session was spent getting to know the group members. This was accomplished through individual introduction stories written from each group member's case history and the information provided in the questionnaire (see Appendix 5D). Prior experiences in therapy were discussed, and group members were invited to share their personal goals for therapy.

Step Three: Discussing the Goals of Treatment (Session 5)

Discussion of the goals of treatment was also accomplished during the first treatment session. The rationale of the treatment, treatment objectives, and treatment format were discussed in the group. Group members were invited to ask questions about the treatment and make suggestions for topics to be covered in the communication notebook. A story format entitled *What Is Cooperative Group Treatment* could also be used to explain the treatment.

Step 4: Treatment Stories (Sessions 6–17)

Introducing the Stories

Following the introductions and explanation of treatment, the first story was introduced and read aloud by the clinician as the group members followed with their copy. One copy was provided to both group members to encourage cooperative skills. Communication notebook pages were reviewed and used with the story. Two to three stories were introduced per topic to allow sufficient use of the new communication notebook material. In this case study, story themes were introduced in the following sequence: (1) me and my family (sessions 4 and 5), (2) maps (sessions 6 and 7), (3) about my stroke (sessions 8 and 9), (4) time (sessions 10 and 11), (5) numbers and money (sessions 12 and 13), (6) common phrases (session 14), (7) hobbies (session 16), (8) foods (session 18), and (9) the home program and discharge (session 18).

Reviewing Key Information in the Story

Each story included five to six comprehension questions designed to target and reinforce the key information in the story (see Appendix 5E). Group members took turns reading the comprehension questions and highlighting the most important words in the question. For example, in one question in Appendix 5E, "What Is Aphasia?" the words *what* and *aphasia* were highlighted in yellow. Next, the group members found the answer to the question in the body of the text and highlight the answer in yellow. The key words in the next comprehension question were highlighted in blue, with the answer also highlighted in blue. This color-coding system aided the group in locating information in the body of the text, if the comprehension question was used as a facilitation cue during the story recall.

Story Recall

After reading and reviewing the story, the group recalled the story as a team, taking turns to share information via any communication modality. Legal sized clipboards with pen and paper were provided for writing or drawing pertinent information. All communications were scored collectively; therefore, group members were encouraged to help each other by cueing omitted information. All responses were scored for content only: Story sequence accuracy was not scored.

Discharge (Session 18)

The discharge session involved the collection of outcome data and the distribution of the home program. To gather outcome data, social validation questionnaires were presented to group members and their spouses (see Appendixes 5B and 5C). Social validation outcome data, progress on treatment stories, and generalization probes were subsequently discussed with the group. Finally, a home program was introduced with a story entitled *How to Complete the Home Program* (see Appendix 5F). The home program, which consisted of two main activities, was accompanied by detailed instructions (see Appendix 5G).

Example of a Typical Session

The following example describes the session that focused on time. Three stories were used to address this topic: *About Time, SV's Tuesday*, and *CB's Schedule*.

After the group had assembled and talked about their weekend activities, the theme of the day was introduced. New communication notebook pages were then reviewed and edited.

The first story, *About Time*, was used to present the overall concept of time and its various uses. The next two stories, *CB's Schedule*, and *SV's Tuesday* were written from information provided by spouses and were designed to aid the group members in communicating their appointments and daily activities to the group. The story *SV's Tuesday* was first read at a moderate pace by the clinician. Each group member then took turns reading and highlighting the key words in the question and answering the question using any communication modality. Group members were encouraged to use the communication notebook during their responses and practiced cueing strategies by answering the questions. Often, group members pointed to the appropriate answer in the story and, with cueing from the clinician, communicated the answer in another modality to expand their communication abilities. The clinician scored the responses in terms of accuracy, promptness, efficiency, and complexity according to a scoring system outlined and in terms of the gist score (see Table 5-1 and Figure 5-1).

Next, the clients recalled the story as completely as possible, taking turns to convey information, while the clinician timed and transcribed the communication on line. Because the communication was scored collectively, the group members were encouraged to help each other if they became stuck. Each group member developed favorite cueing strategies. For example, SV frequently announced her help saying "hey" and gesturing her clue to her partner, and CB tended to point to his clue in the communication book or spell out a word using his alphabet board. After the recall, the clients reviewed the communication transcribed as a team and compared it to the original story.

The next story, *CB's Schedule*, was introduced and followed the same format as the story *About Time*. There was only enough time left to read the new story. Consequently, the comprehension questions and recall were completed during the next session. The session ended by reviewing the improvements made during the hour and reviewing activities for home practice (i.e., using the new communicative notebook pages in a new environment and reviewing or previewing the stories used for that particular topic).

Case Example

CB, a 62-year-old man, had a left-side cerebrovascular accident following a thyroidectomy. During his acute hospital stay, he was diagnosed with aphasia, moderate to severe apraxia of speech, and right-side hemiplegia. He received approximately 3 months of speech-language treatment.

During cooperative group treatment baseline testing, CB achieved an Aphasia Quotient of 66.1 on the Western Aphasia Battery, which falls below the normal range of 93.8 to 100. Results indicated that he had a moderate Broca's aphasia. Reading comprehension was assessed with the Reading Comprehension Battery for Aphasia. This assessment indicated strong reading skills at the single-word and sentence level with impairment at the short-paragraph level. Functional communication skills were assessed using two subtests of the American Speech-Language Hearing Association's Functional Assessment of Communication Skills for Adults. CB received an overall communication independence mean score of 5.45, indicating that he communicated with moderate assistance. During probe testing, CB retold three short stories over three trials at an average rate of 4.1 ipm. He received accuracy scores ranging from 2 to 15, with an average modified PICA percentile score of 5.4 (i.e., comprehensible response but not an attempt at the task item) and an average communicative gist score of 18.4%.

At the beginning of cooperative group treatment, CB frequently appeared hesitant during group story-retelling tasks, leaving his therapy partner to dominate most of the communication. Additionally, he frequently became frustrated while trying to communicate and would state, "I don't know" or "It's hard," and abandon communication. After approximately 2 weeks, he became more assertive during discussions and story-retelling tasks. For example, he began to hold up his hand to signal more time before his partner cued him and started to offer cues himself. Another change occurred in terms of group dynamic. Initially, CB looked primarily to the clinician to run the session, keeping eye contact with his partner at a minimum. As the treatment progressed, many activities became group directed in terms of when to repeat stories, when to add personal adjuncts to the stories, and when to take breaks. Many decisions involved group discussions, before consensus was reached. Eye contact increased between the group members, and group encouragement and support began to evolve. CB became more demonstrative about his needs and wants from the therapy and seemed to take ownership. His visible frustration lessened and his diligence increased as he learned new communication strategies.

Improvement was also noted in group story retelling. By session 17, at the end of a treatment trial, CB retold a short story at a rate of 7.6 ipm, with an average severity score of 11 percentile points (utterances ranging from 7 to 12) and a communicative gist score of 73%. These scores indicated that CB not only increased his attempts of communication during this task but also improved the overall consistency and accuracy of his utterances. In addition, he expanded his communication modalities from only verbal communication to include written, verbal, and gestural modalities. This increase in modalities directly reflected an increase in his communication accuracy and reduction in severity scores.

Post-treatment generalization probes also reflected improvement on the procedural short story, where ipm increased from 3.5 to 12.0 over the 17 sessions. Accuracy and severity scores were inconsistent, as he ranged from the 7.7 percentile (utterances ranged from 5 to 15) at the beginning of the quarter to the 6.5 percentile (ranging from 4 to 12) at the end of the quarter.

Life outside of cooperative therapy also seemed to improve for CB. His wife began to understand that he had the same thoughts, ideas, and interests that he had always had and that his difficulty was in expressing them, not in thinking of them. Her communication with him changed dramatically, as she started to talk to him, give him choices, and allow him to answer for himself.

Results of the social validation questionnaires were encouraging. Both CB and his spouse indicated that they found the treatment valuable and useful, saw increasing use of the communication notebook, and would recommend this treatment to other aphasic individuals. The only change CB stated that he would make would be to change the frequency of the treatment probes from bimonthly to monthly.

Important Points About This Treatment

The following points are important considerations for cooperative group therapy:

• *Group dynamics*. This treatment lends itself to personal growth. Because it is cooperative by design, it fosters team spirit and commitment among team members. Motivation and participation are high throughout almost all of the treatments. Absences and tardiness are rare. Group members share personal information and encourage each other when one becomes frustrated or disheartened.

• *Group size*. This dyad is small enough to effect quantifiable change on treatment tasks; however, it is dynamic enough to preserve the social relevance and functionality of traditional group treatment.

• *Camaraderie*. Group members relate intimately with another person who has similar deficits. This allows them to see another person improve and realize new hope for their own difficulties.

• *Functionality*. This treatment is designed to increase discourse. Conversation is the key element of human interactions. Because these treatment stories were written about the clients' interests, the discourse topics were functional and practical.

Common Questions and Solutions

Question: What if one group member dominates the story retell?

Answer: This problem was rectified in the moderate group treat-
             ment by instructing the group members to take turns
             communicating information during the story retell.
Question: What if one group member does not spontaneously cue his
             or her partner?
Answer: Initially, the clinician should model cueing strategies for
             the clients and request that each client repeat the cue
             provided. Possible cueing strategies are also reviewed
             as the group members read and answer the compre-
             hension questions of the story. As treatment progresses,
             cueing strategies become more natural, as each client
             finds his or her preferred strategies.
Question: How much preparation time did it take to prepare the
             stories and communication book pages?
Answer: Preparation ranged between 1 and 2 hours per week.
             However, now that all of the formats and resources are
             collected, another cooperative group treatment would
             take only one-third of that preparation time.

Recommended Sources for Materials

All the stories for the moderate cooperative group were written by
the clinician from the information in the environmental questionnaire. Visual aids were taken from desktop calendars, atlases, and
textbooks.

References

1. Hux K, Beukelman DR, Garrett KL. Augmentative and Alternative
   Communication for Persons with Aphasia. In R Chapey (ed), Language
   and Intervention Strategies in Adult Aphasia. Baltimore: Williams &
   Wilkins, 1994;338.
2. Kertesz A. Western Aphasia Battery. New York: Grune & Stratton,
   1982.
3. La Pointe L, Horner J. Reading Comprehension Battery of Aphasia.
   Tigard, OR: CC Publications, 1979.
4. Darley FL, Aronson AE, Brown JR. Motor Speech Disorders. Philadelphia: Saunders, 1975.

5. Frattali CM, Thompson CK, Holland AL, et al. American Speech-Language Association Functional Assessment of Communication Skills for Adults. Rockville, MD: ASHA, 1995.
6. Porch B. The Porch Index of Communicative Ability. Austin, TX: PRO-ED, 1981.

Appendix 5A:
Generalization Probes

Restaurant Review (Narrative)

Fat Ed's Hickory Pit
(510) 835-7866

There is a new restaurant in Oakland. It opened 2 months ago. It is owned by Ed Miller and his wife, Lisa. The restaurant is called Fat Ed's Hickory Pit. The restaurant is located in downtown Oakland. The address is 1575 Seventh Street. The restaurant serves barbecue food. Fat Ed's is famous for a chicken dish. A main dish costs between $8.00 and $12.00. Smoking is not allowed. You must call for reservations. (76 words)

Questions:

1. What is the name of the new restaurant in Oakland?

2. What is the address and telephone number?

3. What type of food is served?

4. How much does a main dish cost?

5. What is their smoking policy?

Taking a Bath (Procedural)

A good way to relax is to take a bubble bath. There are several steps to make a bubble bath. First, fill the tub with water. Use hot and cold water to get the perfect temperature. Next, add the bubble bath crystals. When the tub is full of water, undress and climb in. Soak for a while. Now use the soap to clean yourself. Next, rinse off, step out of the tub, and dry yourself. Finally, drain the tub.
(78 words)

Questions:

1. Why do you take a bubble bath?

2. What is the first thing you do?

3. How do you get the perfect temperature?

4. Soak for a while, then _____.

5. What is the last thing you do?

Tree Frogs (Narrative)

There are 26 tree-frog species in North America. There are about 600 worldwide. They are found on the Pacific Coast from Canada to Mexico. The tree frog is 1 to 2 inches long. Its color may be gray, brown, or green. Most live in trees and shrubs. They cling to branches with their sticky feet. Their loud, clear trill is a common sign of spring. It can be heard for over half a mile.
(75 words)

Questions:

1. How many tree frogs are there in the world?

2. The tree frog can be found from _____ to _____.

3. Where do they live?

4. How long is the tree frog?

5. What color(s) is the tree frog?

6. Their trill is a common sign of _____.

Appendix 5B:
Social Validation Questionnaire for Cooperative Group Study: Moderate Group (Patient)

How would you rate your progress in this treatment?

1	2	3	4	5	6	7

Poor   Fair   Excellent

How has this treatment affected your communication in other situations?

1	2	3	4	5	6	7

Not at all   Some   Significantly

How would you rate the therapeutic and communicative value of this treatment?

1	2	3	4	5	6	7

Poor   Fair   Excellent

How would you rate the materials used in this treatment?

1	2	3	4	5	6	7

Poor　　　　　　　　　　　　　　Fair　　　　　　　　　　　　　　Excellent

Would you recommend this treatment to other aphasic individuals?

1	2	3	4	5	6	7

No　　　　　　　　　　　　　　Maybe　　　　　　　　　　　　Yes

How do you rate the value of the communication notebook?

1	2	3	4	5	6	7

Poor　　　　　　　　　　　　　　Fair　　　　　　　　　　　　　　Excellent

How frequently do you anticipate using the communication notebook?

1	2	3	4	5	6	7

Not at all　　　　　　　　　　Occasionally　　　　　　　　Frequently

Which communication type do you feel is most effective for you?

Writing　　　　　　Speech　　　　　　Gestures　　　　　　Combined

Name one thing you liked about this treatment.

Name one thing you would change about this treatment.

Appendix 5C:
Social Validation Questionnaire for Cooperative Group Study: Moderate Group (Spouse)

How would you rate your spouse's progress in this treatment?

1	2	3	4	5	6	7

Poor   Fair   Excellent

How has this treatment affected his/her communication in other situations?

1	2	3	4	5	6	7

Not at all   Some   Significantly

How would you rate the therapeutic and communicative value of this treatment?

1	2	3	4	5	6	7

Poor   Fair   Excellent

How would you rate the materials used in this treatment?

1	2	3	4	5	6	7

Poor   Fair   Excellent

Would you recommend this treatment to other aphasic individuals?

1	2	3	4	5	6	7

No   Maybe   Yes

How do you rate the value of the communication notebook?

1	2	3	4	5	6	7

Poor   Fair   Excellent

How frequently do you anticipate your spouse will use the communication notebook?

1	2	3	4	5	6	7

Not at all   Occasionally   Frequently

Which communication type do you feel is most effective for your spouse?

Writing   Speech   Gestures   Combined

Name one thing you liked about this treatment.

Name one thing you would change.

Appendix 5D: Informational Questionnaire

Cooperative Group Treatment

Personal Information

Name: _____

Name of spouse: _____

Number of siblings: _____

Name(s) of child: _____

Name(s) of grandchild: _____

Who lives in your home with you? _____

Travel

Place of birth: _____

Area(s) where you grew up: _____

Cities where children and grandchildren live: _____

Favorite places to go on vacation: _____

Favorite city(ies) in the United States: _____

Favorite city or country in the world: _____

Places traveled abroad: _____

Travel wish (if you could go anywhere for a visit, where would you go):

_____

Entertainment

Favorite hobbies before the stroke: _____

Current hobbies and interests: _____

Favorite sport: _____

Favorite television show: _____

Favorite movie: _____

Favorite actor or actress: _____

Favorite restaurant: _____

Favorite type of food: _____

Most disliked food: _____

Are you a member of a club or organization? If so which one(s)? __

_____

Favorite type of music: _____

Most disliked type of music: _____

Appendix 5E:
Stories, Visual Aids, and Communication Notebook Inserts Used to Introduce the Topic "About My Stroke"*

What Is Aphasia?

Aphasia is a disruption in understanding and using language.

Most cases of aphasia occur after a stroke.

A stroke is the result of either too much or no blood to the brain.

Persons with aphasia have not lost their language.

But, have lost the ability to recall and use language.

There are physical problems that occur with aphasia.

Most common is a weakness or paralysis in the right arm or leg.

These symptoms usually improve over time.

(78 words)

---

*The figures in this appendix are reproduced with permission from R Love, W Webb. Neurology for the Speech-Language Pathologist (3rd ed). Boston: Butterworth–Heinemann, 1996.

Questions

1. What is aphasia?
2. What is the most common cause of aphasia?
3. A stroke is the result of _____.
4. Have persons with aphasia lost their language?
5. What are common physical problems associated with aphasia?

About Our Strokes

CB had a stroke on April 29, 1992.

That was 4 years ago.

The stroke followed an operation on his thyroid.

Which resulted in damage to the front, left side of his brain.

This caused an aphasia and a speech disorder called apraxia.

SV's stroke was on November 18, 1991.

That was 4 and one-half years ago.

Her stroke caused damage in the front, left side of her brain.

Which also resulted in an aphasia and apraxia.

(76 words)

Questions

1. When was CB's stroke?
2. Where was the damage?
3. This caused an _____ and _____.
4. When was SV's stroke?
5. Where was the damage?

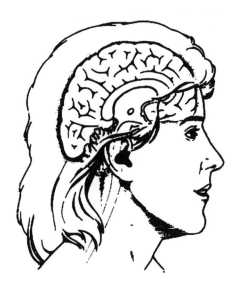

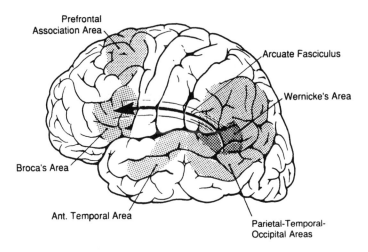

Figure A5E-1. Illustrations for communication notebook to accompany stroke stories.

Sample Communication Notebook Pages to Accompany the Stroke Stories

November 18, 1991

Stroke ⇒	Brain damage (left side)
Aphasia ⇒	Difficulty using and understanding language (does not affect intelligence)
Apraxia ⇒	Difficulty moving speech muscles to make sounds

Can communicate, just takes longer

You can help by:

- Giving me more time
- Being patient
- Giving me the chance
- Looking at me when you talk
- Slowing down when you talk

Appendix 5F:
Example of Story Used to
Introduce the Home Program

How to Complete the Home Program (Procedural)

A home program is a way to review and maintain what you have learned in therapy. Try to practice every other day for 30 minutes.

First find the envelope marked *stories*. Choose a story you want to work on and find the matching audio tape. Read the story as you listen to the tape. Work through the questions. Use a highlighter pen to find the most important information. Find the answer to the question in the story. Next, practice recalling the information in the story to a partner. Check the story to see which components you remembered. Next, find the pile of index cards. Take turns communicating the idea on the index card to your partner without showing him or her the card. (123 words)

Questions:

1. What is a home program?

2. How often should you practice?

3. What is the first thing you do?

4. Find the answer to the question in the _____.

5. Who do you recall the story with?

6. What do you do with the index cards?

Appendix 5G:
Home Program

General Directions

You have worked hard and made some noticeable gains in therapy. Home practice is an important way of reviewing and maintaining what you have learned in therapy. All the activities will follow those we have done in the clinic. Try to choose a time during the day when you are the least tired and practice in a quiet place. Each practice session should take place every other day and last approximately 30 minutes. It is not necessary to work on all tasks each session; however, please alternate the activities you choose to work on. For example, if you work on listening and reading comprehension one day, be sure to work on story recall and charades the following session.

Specific Instructions

It is important to keep track of your work. Please put all of your papers into the notebook provided. This will allow you to review your progress. When communicating during the tasks or in your everyday conversations, use any communication modality: notebook, gestures, speech, or writing. Try to use as many modalities as you can. Your progress in therapy has shown that your communication increases when you combine your approaches. In other words, you have a better chance of being understood when you communicate using gestures and speech, rather than just speech. If you are having trouble with a word or concept, stop, take a breath, and try again. It may help to think of another way to communicate your thought, using either a different modality (e.g., gesture or writing) or a different description. Take your time and remember you know the information, it just takes longer to communicate it.

Directions to Spouse

Encourage your spouse to use his notebook and gestures whenever possible. Try not to anticipate his needs, but wait until at least one attempt is given. If he uses phrases such as "I don't know" or "It's too hard," encourage him to keep going and find another way to communicate (e.g., notebook, gestures, writing). Help reinforce his efforts. When you see him use alternate methods of communication, comment on his progress and offer support.

Listening and Reading Comprehension

This task is designed as a review and follow-up on the work we have done in therapy. In the envelope marked *stories*, you will find eight short stories followed by four to six comprehension questions. In your packet you will also find eight, 2-minute audio cassettes that match the stories. Find the tape to match the story you want to work on. Listen to the tape as you read your story. Work through the questions one at a time. Using a highlighter pen, mark the most important words in the questions to help you summarize the information. Find the answer to the question in the body of the text and mark the answer with the highlighter. When you have finished, you may check your answers with the answer sheet provided. You may work on the stories in any order after you have completed the one marked *How to complete the home program*.

When you tire of the stories provided, you can find your own stories in a newspaper or magazine. Try to keep the stories to about 75 words. Work through the story and highlight the most important information.

I Am Hungry	I Am Cold

Figure 5G-1. Examples of charade activity cards.

Story Recall

After you have read a story and worked through the comprehension questions, turn over the story and practice recalling the information to a partner. Use your communication notebook, gestures, speech, and writing to get your point across to your listener. Take about 2–3 minutes to complete this task, then turn over your page and go over the story, marking which key components you communicated and which ones to remember for next time. This task is designed to help you practice communicating information about yourself and information you have read or experienced. The more you practice communicating, the more automatic it will become.

Modified Charades

This activity is designed to be played in pairs. In the envelope marked *charades* you will find a pile of 20 index cards. On each index card is a word or idea to communicate to your partner. Anyway you can, without showing your partner the card, communicate the message so that your partner will guess what is written on your card. Take turns drawing a card from the pile. The messages on the cards are items that you may frequently need to communicate. There is a separate stack of blank cards for you to add other phrases and ideas to the pile. Remember, this is your therapy. Feel free to add things that you feel are relevant. Examples of two messages are in Figure 5G-1.

6

Other Cooperative Learning Methods

Jan Avent

In Chapters 1–5, cooperative group treatment and variations of this treatment are discussed. The purpose of this chapter is to focus on other cooperative learning methods and describe how these methods could be adapted for aphasia group treatment. The first goal is to discuss how to modify many aphasia group treatment tasks to create cooperative learning opportunities. The second goal is to outline various cooperative learning methods that could be adapted to aphasia group treatment. These methods are used in academic settings but hold promise as viable group treatments with appropriate modifications.

Modifying Group Tasks to Become Cooperative Activities

Simply putting clients together in a group does not ensure cooperative interactions.[1, 2] For a group to be cooperative, the members must interact, have equal participation, be interdependent on team members, and be accountable for their learning and contributions.[3] Using these characteristics, many aphasia group activities can be modified to become a cooperative learning activity. The following guidelines are helpful when structuring a cooperative activity:[4]

- To capitalize on clients' intrinsic motivations, cooperative tasks should be relevant and important to the group members.[4]

- Cooperative tasks should be designed to provide opportunities for group members to work collaboratively through social interaction.

- The goals for cooperative tasks should be broad or open-ended enough to allow a group to complete a task in a way that it finds beneficial. Open-ended tasks encourage group members to be more autonomous.

- Activities that lend themselves to cooperative tasks are those that require multiple viewpoints and shared responsibility. Cooperative activities are those in which each group member can make meaningful contributions to the group. In the best cooperative groups, partners complement each other.

An easy way to try a cooperative learning task is to begin with a simple collaboration. During the activity, provide repeated opportunities to learn cooperative skills, and give the group members an opportunity to evaluate the activity.[4]

Collaboration

The more enjoyable the task, the easier it is for the group to work cooperatively. Collaboration includes team building, respecting different opinions, and providing positive feedback. Often, team-building exercises, such as sharing information about each group member, build on the skill of equal participation. For example, the clinician should have each person say one thing about himself or herself during introductions. Polling group members on opinions about current events also fosters a respect for different points of view. Another method for promoting collaboration is to practice interviewing skills. As each person practices answering interview questions, the other members are instructed to provide promotive or positive feedback about each person's performance.

Opportunities to Learn Cooperative Skills

Many traditional individual treatment goals, such as naming or writing tasks, can be modified to teach groups about cooperation. For example, in a group of three clients with a goal of improved writing skills, one client dictates a list of words, while the other two clients write the words. Following dictation, the clients check their answers for errors, correct any errors, and turn in the dictation to the clinician for a group accuracy score. The clients alternate the role of providing dictation and checking the answers.

Evaluating Benefits

Following all activities, the members are given opportunities to evaluate the benefits of working together with a social validation questionnaire. These evaluations can be done through rating scales or group discussions about the beneficial aspects of treatment. Often, the members use the evaluation opportunity to take more responsibility for the direction and content of their treatment.

Example of Cooperative Learning Activities

There are many examples from the cooperative learning literature of cooperative learning tasks that are used in academic settings. These activities are designed to enhance the acquisition of information and provide students opportunities to work on their interactional skills. Examples of these different methods and the recommended number of members per group are shown in Table 6-1. Each method is described separately in this section and is followed by suggested activities for aphasia groups.

Jigsaw

Description

The jigsaw group consists of two to four members. Members in a group read different sections of the same stimulus materials. For example, in a

Table 6-1. Examples of Cooperative Learning Methods and the Recommended Number of Members Per Group

Cooperative Learning Method	Number of Members Per Group
Jigsaw[5]	2–4
Jigsaw II[6]	3–4
Scripted cooperation[8]	2
Peer editing[9]	2–4
Cooperative integrated reading and composition[6]	2
Drill-review pairs[9]	2
Student teams: achievement divisions[6]	4–5
Q (question)-approach[11]	3–4

group of three individuals, one person reads about the Monarch butterfly, the second reads about the migration patterns of Monarch butterflies, and the third reads about plants that attract Monarch butterflies. Comprehension of the entire article depends on each member of the group teaching the other members about his or her specific topic.[5]

Suggested Adaptations for Aphasia Groups

Mild Groups
Each client in the group reads different sections from a *Time* magazine article and answers pertinent questions provided by the clinician about his or her section. Each client then takes turns summarizing the information from his or her section, using the clinician's questions to cover the essential information. The process continues until the entire article has been discussed.

Moderate Groups
The clinician prepares an itinerary for a trip and divides the route among the group members so that each person has a portion of the trip. To describe the starting place, route, and destination, each person provides his or her information by using maps, gestures, drawings, verbalizations, or any combination of these.

Severe Groups
With a group of three clients, the clinician presents stacks of noun cards, verb cards, and object cards. One client selects a card from the noun card

stack, the next client selects a card from the verb stack, and the last client selects a card from the object stack. The task is to put the cards in the correct order to make a sentence. For example, one card may read "the man," the second may read "is eating," and the third "the apple." The clients put their cards down in order, and the clinician provides pictures of each word above the card. If the sentence is in error, the clinician asks the group members to check their answer and agree on the correct order.

Jigsaw II

Description

The jigsaw II group consists of three to four members per group with three to four different groups for a total of nine to 16 members. Members assigned to each group read the same stimulus material. Although each member reads the same story, each person has a different set of questions to answer at the end of the reading. Members from different groups form new groups to discuss the same topic or questions. Following this discussion, the original groups reconvene, so that each member can teach his or her teammates about the material.[6]

Suggested Adaptation for Aphasia Groups

Mild Groups

In a group of nine clients, smaller groups of three members each are formed. Each of the nine clients reads a short, three-page mystery story from the *Five Minute Mysteries*.[7] After the story is completed, one person in each of the three-member groups receives questions to answer from the beginning of the story, the second person in each of the smaller groups receives questions from the middle of the story, and the third person in each of the smaller groups answers questions from the end of the story. Next, the clients who received questions from the beginning of the story form a group to discuss the answers, those who received questions from the middle of the story meet together, and those receiving questions from the end of the story meet together. After the questions are answered in each group, the original groups reconvene. The members discuss each of their sections and solve the mystery.

Moderate Groups

The set-up of moderate groups is similar to the mild group: Nine members are divided into three smaller groups. Each client is given a procedural story that is out of order; the clinician reads the misordered story to the group. After the story is read, one person in each group is asked to select the first one to two steps in the procedures; the second client selects the next two steps; and the third client selects the last two steps. The selections are not discussed at this stage. Next, the clients who chose the first two steps form a group to discuss their selections, those who chose the next two steps meet together, and those who chose the last two steps meet together. After the discussions, the original groups reconvene to put the procedural story in the proper sequence.

Severe Groups

The task of severe groups is similar to moderate-group tasks. With severe groups, picture sequence cards are used to determine the beginning, middle, and end of a story in the sequence. Members are divided into two to three smaller groups of three members each. Each client is given the same set of six sequence cards that depict a story. One person in each group is selected to find the first two pictures in the sequence (beginning of story); the second person selects the next two pictures (middle of story); and the third person selects the last two pictures (end of story). Next, the clients who were assigned the beginning of the story form a group to decide on the first two pictures, those who received the middle portion meet together, and those who received the final story assignment meet together. After the groups select their portions, the clinician reviews the selections and assists the groups if errors exist. After review, the original groups reconvene. The members put their stories in the proper sequence.

Scripted Cooperation

Description

The scripted cooperation group consists of two members. Scripted cooperation is designed to provide a model of effective skills in learning about new information. It can be applied to a variety of tasks, including writing, procedural discourse, and narrative discourse. The text is divided into smaller units. Both partners read the same unit. The first partner retells the first unit information without looking at the text. The second partner provides feedback, adds information, and corrects errors. Both partners discuss the information and briefly review the previous story elements adding the most recent information and relating it to prior knowledge. Both partners read the next section, and the partners switch roles for the new unit. The process continues until the passage is read.[8]

Suggested Adaptation for Aphasia Groups

Mild Groups
The clinician asks the clients to select a travel destination. Using a travel guide, clients take turns reading paragraphs about places to visit, lodgings, and restaurants. The client who reads the paragraph then paraphrases the paragraph, as the partner verifies the information. Following the completion of the reading, the clients list hotels from three price categories (i.e., expensive, moderate, and economical), a variety of restaurants to try, and various sites to visit (e.g., museums).

Moderate Groups
Using short sentences and illustrations for the instructions, the clients take turns teaching each other how to play a board or card game. The partners read the first instruction, and one client demonstrates the instruction. The partner verifies the accuracy of the demonstration. The roles are alternated until all of the rules have been explained.

Severe Groups
In a previous session, the clients pick an activity for the next session (e.g., getting coffee at a local restaurant). The clinician prepares a story about the activity using single words, pictures, and drawings. The clients review the story with the clinician and take turns communicating where they will go, what they will buy, and how much it will cost. In the paraphrasing portion of the story, the communicator has the option of using words, picture cards, drawings, or gestures to indicate where, what, and how much. The partner uses the clinician-generated story to verify the information.

Peer Editing

Description

The peer editing group consists of two to four members. This approach is designed for writing tasks. The members in a group are assigned a writing task. Each member describes what he or she is planning to write. Other members ask questions and help outline the sequence. The group members work together to get each person's first paragraph written. Members then complete their written assignment individually. When the writing assignment is completed, the group members proofread each other's response. The members rewrite their papers based on group feedback. The group members again proofread the papers and turn them in.[9]

Suggested Adaptation for Aphasia Groups

Mild Groups

The group watches a 20-minute videotaped segment of a news show. Following the viewing, the members discuss the gist of the segment, while the clinician compiles a list of the essential information. The group then decides how to start a written account of the show. Each person begins with the same sentence: *This show was about....* For the next 15 minutes, each person writes an account of the story. Next, the clients trade papers and edit for spelling, content, and grammatical errors. When the paper is returned, each person rewrites his or her paper making the appropriate corrections.

Moderate Groups

Each client in the group is given a story framework about his or her life history. For example, the framework includes incomplete sentences, such as *I was born...*, and the client selects a response from a list of phrases (e.g., *in Cleveland*). Each person completes the story. The clients then trade stories to verify accuracy and spelling. Answer sheets are provided for the partners. Next, the stories are returned for corrections.

Severe Groups

A story about each client's family is used to work on family members' names. A family tree with photographs is provided for each client. Under each picture, the first letter of each name, along with blanks for the remaining letters, is provided (e.g., *J _ _* for *Joe*). A list of family names is available for copying. Each client completes his or her family tree and then exchanges stories for editing by another group member. Answers are provided for each editor for verification. Stories are returned for correction.

Cooperative Integrated Reading and Composition

Description

Cooperative integrated reading and comprehension groups consist of two members per group with one to eight different groups for a total of two to sixteen members. It is designed to work on reading, writing, and oral language in a cooperative framework. A series of activities are used to reinforce the comprehension and verbal retelling of a particular story. First, the teacher describes the story, leads a discussion about the story, and reviews new vocabulary words. After the stories are introduced, the members are given a story packet to work on in their group. After reading the story silently, the partners take turns reading the story. Next, the members are given questions about the story to answer, which regard elements such as the topic, the characters, and the setting. The members are then given a list of important vocabulary words to practice saying aloud. The next task is to assign word meanings to the vocabulary words by matching the appropriate definition to each vocabulary word. Next, the partners practice retelling the story using their vocabulary words.[6]

Suggested Adaptation for Aphasia Groups

Mild Groups
The members are given a movie review to discuss. Pertinent information about where the film takes place, its time frame, and actors are reviewed. In small groups of two to three clients, the group reads the review and answers questions about it. The group practices saying the important vocabulary words aloud and gives each other feedback about their verbal productions. Following the verbal vocabulary practice, the vocabulary words are matched with their definition. The last task is to paraphrase the review using the vocabulary words.

Moderate Groups
The clinician provides short descriptions of two local restaurants. The group reads the descriptions and answers questions about the location, type of food, hours, and prices. Next, the group practices saying the answers to the questions. Following the verbal practice, the members match the information to the appropriate restaurant. After the matching task, the clients indicate which restaurant they would like to try.

Severe Groups
The group is given five current-event pictures for a question-and-answer discussion. For example, the topic might be world leaders. Photographs with names of the leaders of five countries are shown. Maps are used to locate each country. The clients then practice matching each photograph with the appropriate country name or map location. Next, the members practice copying the name of each leader and drawing a line to the appropriate listed country. Following the practice, the clinician asks the group to match the leader to a world map.

Drill-Review Pairs

Description

The drill-review pair group consists of two members per group with any number of groups participating. The group members are given a packet of problems to solve. The first partner reads the first problem and explains the procedure for solving it. The second partner checks or critiques the explanation. The second partner then reads the next problem and explains the procedure for solving this second problem, and the first partner checks the explanation. When all of the problems have been solved, the procedures are reviewed with the teacher.[9]

Suggested Adaptation for Aphasia Groups

Mild Groups

The group is given a packet of short paragraphs and asked to determine the topic of each short story. The first partner reads the first paragraph, identifies the topic, and explains why it is the topic. The second partner checks the answer and critiques the explanation. For the next paragraph, the roles are reversed.

Moderate Groups

The first partner is given a short sentence to read and find the misspelled word. Once the misspelled word is located, the word is spelled correctly by writing it above the misspelled word. The second partner verifies the answer. Then, the second partner reads the next sentence, finds the misspelled word, and corrects it. The first partner then verifies the answer.

Severe Groups

The group is given a packet of pictures of well-known pairs (e.g., salt and pepper or baseball and bat). These are reviewed by the clinician. Next, the first partner is given either a matched pair (e.g., squirrel and nut) or a mismatched pair (e.g., coffee and hand lotion). The task is to indicate whether the pair is a match. If the pair is not matched, a picture of the appropriate pair must be located from a pile of picture pairs. The second partner verifies the answer. For the next picture pair, the roles are reversed.

Student Teams: Achievement Divisions

Description

The achievement division student teams consist of four to five members with two to three different groups for a total of eight to fifteen members. The teacher prepares a stimulus packet of pictures, math problems, directions, reading materials, and so on. He or she also provides worksheets about the content. The teacher states the objectives for the materials and provides worksheets so that the teams can master the information. During the team study, the members are to learn the material and help their teammates learn the material. They are given only two worksheets, thereby forcing them to work together to answer the questions. There are basic ground rules for the group work: (1) The members are responsible for making sure everyone practices the material, (2) no one is finished practicing until all the teammates have mastered the material, (3) members should ask teammates before asking the teacher (i.e., "ask three before you ask me"), (4) the teacher should have teammates explain answers to each other, and (5) the worksheets are used for practice not just for filling out. Once the group has practiced together, the members discuss the information with the teacher.[6]

Suggested Adaptation for Aphasia Groups

Mild Groups

An educational card game, such the American History Quiz,[10] could be used along with content information from a history book or the Internet. The clients take turns asking questions from the quiz card. For example, a quiz about the Alamo includes questions like *In what Texas city is the Alamo located?* or *From what nation did the Texans revolt in 1835?* All answers are discussed and agreed on before asking the next question. Any unanswered questions are looked up in a reference source. Once all questions are answered, the group practices asking and answering questions. Finally, the clinician asks the quiz-card questions for the group to answer.

Moderate Groups

The group is given a *TV Guide* and questions to answer about their favorite television shows. For example, sample questions include *Are* ER *and* Chicago Hope *televised on the same night?* or *Does* David Letterman *come on at 9 o'clock?* Once the questions are answered, the clients take turns practicing the answers. After the practice period, the clinician asks the group the questions.

Severe Groups
The clinician provides a stack of pictures showing number, size, or temperature information. For each appropriate picture, the clinician uses gestures to ask (1) how many? (2) is it big or little? or (3) is it hot or cold? The clients practice gesturing the answers to each other. Following the practice, the clinician asks the group the appropriate question for each picture.

Q (Question)-Approach

Description

The Q-approach group consists of three to four members. The Q-approach is designed to help students learn to generate questions. Two different "question dials" (Q-dials) are used to generate one of the 36 possible questions that are generated by six words on each dial. One pie-shaped dial contains the words *where*, *when*, *who*, *why*, *how*, and *what*. The other dial contains the words *would*, *will*, *might*, *is*, *did*, and *can*. The group is given a topic to discuss with the goal of generating questions about the topic. Each member takes a turn spinning the two question dials to come up with the beginning of a question (e.g., Where would...? or Who is...?). After generating a specified number of questions, the group picks one question to answer using resource materials.[11]

Suggested Adaptation for Aphasia Groups

Mild Groups
During a discussion about current events, each person in the group takes turns asking questions based on the Q–dial approach. Two stacks of cards representing the two dials are used to provide the first two words of a question. Following the question, the group discusses the answer.

Moderate Groups
A stack of pictures depicting a variety of who, what, where, when, why, and how information are used. In groups of two clients, one person has a list of the questions and the other person has a list of answers

for each picture. The clients take turns asking a question and answering the question.

Severe Groups
For severe groups, a stack of pictures like the set used for moderate groups (see "Moderate Groups" above) is used. In groups of two clients, one person points to the printed word *who, when,* or *where.* The partner uses the picture to point to the answer. The roles are reversed for the next question and answer.

References

1. Avent JR. Group treatment in aphasia using cooperative learning method. J Med Speech-Lang Pathol 1997;5:9.
2. Johnson DW, Johnson RT. Learning Together. In S Sharan (ed), Handbook of Cooperative Learning Methods. Westport, CT: Greenwood, 1994;51.
3. Kagan S, Kagan M. The Structural Approach: Six Keys to Cooperative Learning. In S Sharan (ed), Handbook of Cooperative Learning Methods. Westport, CT: Greenwood, 1994;115.
4. Watson M, Solomon D, Dasho S, et al. CDP Cooperative Learning: Working Together to Construct Social, Ethical, and Intellectual Understanding. In S Sharan (ed), Handbook of Cooperative Learning Methods. Westport, CT: Greenwood, 1994;137.
5. Aronson E, Blaney N, Stephan C, et al. The Jigsaw Classroom. Beverly Hills, CA: Sage, 1978.
6. Slavin RE. Cooperative Learning (2nd ed). Boston: Allyn & Bacon, 1995.
7. Weber K. Five-Minute Mysteries. Philadelphia: Running Press, 1989.
8. O'Donnell AM, Dansereau DF. Scripted Cooperation in Student Dyads: A Method for Analyzing and Enhancing Academic Learning and Performance. In R Hertz-Lazarowitz, N Miller (eds), Interaction in Cooperative Groups: The Theoretical Anatomy of Group Learning. New York: Cambridge University Press, 1992;120.
9. Johnson DW, Johnson RT, Smith KA. Cooperative Learning: Increasing College Faculty Instructional Productivity. Washington, DC: George Washington University, 1991.
10. American History Quiz: An Educational Card Game. Smithsonian Institution, 1988.
11. Wiederhold C, Kagan S. Cooperative Questioning and Critical Thinking. In N Davidson, T Worsham (eds), Enhancing Thinking Through Cooperative Learning. New York: Teachers College Press, 1992;198.

Index